TREATMENT OF SUBSTANCE USE DISORDERS

Edited by

Kevin A. Sevarino, M.D., PH.D.

BRUNNER-ROUTLEDGE
New York • London

Published in 2002 by
Brunner-Routledge
29 West 35th Street
New York, NY 10001

Published in Great Britain by
Brunner-Routledge
27 Church Road
Hove, East Sussex, BN3 2FA

1003104937

Brunner-Routledge is an imprint of the Taylor & Francis Group.

Printed in the United States of America on acid-free paper.

10 9 8 7 6 5 4 3 2 1

Library of Congress Cataloging-in-Publication Data
Treatment of substance use disorders / edited by Kevin A. Sevarino
    p. ; cm.— (Key readings in addiction psychiatry)
   Includes bibliographical references and index.
   ISBN 0-415-93362-5 (pbk.)
   1. Substance abuse. 2. Substance abuse—Treatment.   I. Sevarino, Kevin Allen.
II. Series.
   [DNLM: 1. Substance-Related Disorders—therapy—Collected Works. WM 270
T78437 2002]

RC564 .T745 2002
616.86′062—dc21

2002018453

Treatment of Substance Use Disorders

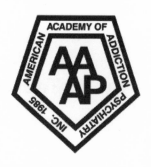

American Academy of Addiction Psychiatry
Key Readings in Addiction Psychiatry

Contents

Introduction to the Key Readings in Addiction Psychiatry Series

The American Academy of Addiction Psychiatry is pleased to announce a new book series entitled Key Readings in Addiction Psychiatry. Substance abuse adversely affects a very large portion of the world's population, causing more deaths, illnesses, and disabilities than any other preventable health condition. According to Dr. Alan I. Leshner (1999), former Director of the National Institute on Drug Abuse, "addiction has so many dimensions and disrupts so many aspects of an individual's life, treatment for this illness is never simple." [1] Scientific advances are occurring at an increasingly rapid rate, leading to an array of effective pharmacologic and behavioral treatment approaches. These new advances are stimulating a new level of scientific curiosity and research and accelerating the application of scientific findings in the clinical setting.

By means of the compilations of up-to-date articles on various aspects of substance use disorders, the American Academy of Addiction Psychiatry, through the Key Readings series, seeks to

- advance the knowledge of those committed to the treatment of substance abuse
- introduce those new to the field of addictions to recent advances in the treatment and prevention of substance use disorders
- inspire those without knowledge of substance use disorders and reinvigorate those with a nihilistic view of their treatment to work to advance the field of addictions beyond its current knowledge base.

Each book will serve as a quick guide to research studies and treatment approaches in the addiction field. They will serve as reference tools, edited by

1. Leshner, A. I. (1999). Principles of Drug Addiction Treatment. National Institute on Drug Abuse, Bethesda, MD.

an expert in the field, keeping today's busy professional informed of timely, critical, and interesting research and clinical treatment issues. Each book within the series will present outstanding articles from leading clinical journals of relevance to the addiction professional whether in clinical, research, administrative, or academic roles. The Key Readings in Addiction Psychiatry series will be presented in several volumes focused on treatment, dual diagnosis, pharmacologic, and psychosocial therapies.

A new book in the series will be published each year, providing a continuous flow of new information in a handy, easily accessible form. This compilation of key readings in one source will be an excellent supplement to textbooks and can be used not only to keep up with rapid change in our field but also in preparation for addiction certification or recertification examinations.

Stephen L. Dilts, M.D., Ph.D.
Past President
American Academy of Addiction Psychiatry

Introduction to Treatment of Substance Use Disorders

This volume, the first in the Key Readings in Addiction Psychiatry series, offers a look at the most up-to-date reviews in the treatment of substance abuse through the use of journal source materials. The readings focus on the "big four" : alcohol (and benzodiazepines), opiates, cocaine, and nicotine. Repeated use and misuse of these substances account for the major portion of adverse economic, medical, and social consequences of substance use disorders. A grounding in the treatment of addiction to these substances will leave the reader well-armed to explore treatment of the many other abused agents, including cannabis, amphetamines, barbiturates, and club drugs such as MDMA.

This compilation begins with three articles dealing with substance use disorders in general. The first two, *Medications for Alcohol, Illicit Drug, and Tobacco Dependence: An Update of Research Findings* by Litten and Allen and *The Pharmacotherapy of Relapse Prevention Using Anticonvulsants* by Kosten, describe the current state of pharmacotherapies for those in active and maintenance phases, respectively, of substance abuse treatment. Pharmacotherapy for substance abuse, delivered in the absence of concomitant behavioral therapy, is notoriously ineffective. *Current Developments in Psychosocial Treatments of Alcohol and Substance Abuse* by Siqueland and Crits-Christoph describes current nonpharmacological approaches to substance use disorders. Subsequent articles are meant to complement the general reviews. *Drug Therapy for Alcohol Dependence* by Swift and *Alcoholism Treatment and Medical Care Costs from Project MATCH* by Holder, Cisler, Longabaugh, Stout, Treno, and Zweben focus on the latest approaches to alcohol-dependence treatment. As alcohol-dependent individuals very commonly become addicted to benzodiazepines, *Use of Anticonvulsants in Benzodiazepine Withdrawal* by Pages and Ries is presented next. This review addresses the most common issue for the sedative/hypnotic-addicted individual: the need for detoxification.

Pharmacological Treatment of Heroin-Dependent Patients by O'Connor and Fiellin and *Methadone vs. L-alpha-acetylmethadol (LAAM) in the Treatment of Opiate Addiction: A Meta-Analysis of the Randomized, Controlled Trials* by Glanz, Klawansky, McAuliffe, and Chalmers provide the latest in treatment of the opiate-dependent individual. Because pharmacotherapies for cocaine dependence are notoriously ineffective, *Old Psychotherapies for Cocaine Dependence Revisited* by Carroll is presented next to review the most up-to-date and frequently used treatment approaches for cocaine addiction. Finally, *New Treatments for Smoking Cessation* by Hughes addresses nicotine dependence. Cigarette smoking is largely ignored or tolerated by the medical community as the "least of his/her problems," but the massive economic and medical consequences of tobacco use logically cannot be ignored any longer.

It is hoped that this compendium of articles will impart to the reader a new appreciation of treatment approaches to substance use disorders and leave all in the field excited by the prospect for new treatment developments.

Kevin A. Sevarino, M.D., Ph.D.
Assistant Professor in Psychiatry
University of Connecticut School of Medicine
and
Co-Chair, Publications and Products Committee
American Academy of Addiction Psychiatry

Chapter 1

Medications for Alcohol, Illicit Drug, and Tobacco Dependence

An Update of Research Findings

Raye Z. Litten, Ph.D.
John P. Allen, Ph.D.

INTRODUCTION

A variety of physiological, psychological, and social factors underlie dependence on psychoactive substances that include alcohol, illicit drugs, and tobacco. While a variety of psychosocial interventions have been developed to assist in resolving these problems, until the past decade or so, little research was undertaken to develop medications that could also assist in treatment of chemically dependent patients. Several medications now appear promising and are likely to significantly influence clinical practice in the future. This article summarizes the state of the knowledge on this topic.

PHARMACOTHERAPY FOR ALCOHOLISM

Progress in development of medications to prevent or reduce drinking is most strikingly illustrated by consideration of two agents, naltrexone and acamprosate. Both have been demonstrated as efficacious and both are currently available for clinical use in a large number of countries. In this section we review research on these agents as well as on disulfiram and the antidepressants fluoxetine and sertraline.

1

Naltrexone

In December 1994, the opioid antagonist naltrexone (Revia) was approved by the U.S. Food and Drug Administration (FDA) as an adjunct to treatment of alcoholism. Since then, it has been approved in 18 additional countries. Approval of naltrexone was based primarily on two landmark studies (O'Malley & Volpicelli). In the first project, 70 alcohol-dependent male outpatients, recruited from a Veterans Affairs (VA) hospital, were treated with either 50 mg of naltrexone or placebo daily for 3 months (Volpicelli, Alterman, Hayashida, & O'Brien, 1992). Patients also received 4 weeks of intensive abstinence-oriented verbal therapy followed by 8 weeks of aftercare treatment. Those on naltrexone experienced fewer drinking days, were less likely to relapse to heavy drinking, and reported lower craving for alcohol.

In the second investigation (O'Malley et al., 1992), male and female alcohol-dependent patients were treated with 50 mg of naltrexone or placebo daily for 3 months. Again, naltrexone was found to reduce both frequency and quantity of drinking. Interestingly, O'Malley and her colleagues also employed two types of psychosocial intervention and observed a difference in treatment outcome as a conjoint function of drug condition and nature of psychosocial treatment. Subjects treated with naltrexone and supportive therapy emphasizing total abstinence achieved the highest rate of abstinence. Those treated with naltrexone and coping skills therapy were less likely to relapse to heavy drinking if they did sample alcohol.

Two recently completed studies have indicated that patient compliance is an important component in naltrexone treatment. In a replication of their first naltrexone study, but with non-VA alcoholic males and females and receiving less intense psychosocial intervention, Volpicelli et al. (1997) reported generally modest effects for assignment to naltrexone in reducing number of days drinking and proclivity to relapse to excessive drinking. Nevertheless, among compliant patients (i.e., those who took medication or placebo at least 90% of the time), naltrexone appeared quite effective. Naltrexone-compliant patients drank on 3% of study days, while equally compliant placebo patients drank on 11% of study days. More than half of the placebo-compliant patients returned to heavy drinking, contrasted with only 14% of the naltrexone-compliant group. No differences in drinking outcome measures emerged between less compliant naltrexone- and placebo-treated groups.

Chick et al. (Litten & Fertig, 1996) completed a 3-month trial of naltrexone in the United Kingdom. Following detoxification, alcohol-abusing and alcohol-dependent patients received either 50 mg of naltrexone or placebo daily in the context of traditional outpatient therapy. Although neither frequency nor quantity of drinking distinguished the groups, patients who remained in the study and were adjudged compliant on the basis of correct pill count on at least 80% of return visits benefitted from naltrexone. The naltrexone-compliant group experienced a 40% decrease in number of drinking days and a 50%

reduction in total number of drinks consumed. In addition, they reported less craving for alcohol than did the compliant placebo-treated group.

In a safety trial with naltrexone administered up to 1 year, the agent appeared well tolerated and nonelicitive of severe adverse effects. The most common side effects were nausea and headaches (Croop, Faulkner, & Labriola, 1997; Litten). In addition, there was no evidence of hepatic injury, an important finding since both alcohol and naltrexone are metabolized by the liver.

To explore the possibility that other opioid antagonists might also aid in reducing drinking, Litten and Fertig (1996) conducted a 3-month, placebo-controlled trial with the opioid antagonist nalmefene. Results of the study indicated that patients treated with nalmefene were less prone to return to heavy drinking than were placebo-treated subjects. Thus, it appears that opioid antagonists other than naltrexone may also have promise in reducing drinking.

Acamprosate

Encouraged by earlier studies suggesting efficacy of acamprosate (Campral) for alcoholic patients (Gerra et al., 1992; Lhuintre et al., 1985, 1990), Lipha Pharmaceuticals recently conducted 11 independent multisite double-blind, placebo-controlled studies in nine European countries, recruiting over 4,000 alcohol-dependent patients. Analyses of pooled data indicated that alcohol-dependent patients treated with acamprosate for 6 to 12 months enjoyed abstinence rates, on average, twice those of placebo-treated patients (Mann, Chabac, Lehert, Potgieter, & Sass, 1995).

Several of the country-specific studies have recently been published. Paille et al. (1995) conducted a 31-site trial of acamprosate with 538 alcohol-dependent patients in France. Subjects were administered either 1.3 g or 2.0 g of acamprosate or placebo daily and also were given traditional supportive psychotherapy. Following 1 year of treatment, both acamprosate groups revealed higher rates of continuous sobriety (significant at 6 months, but not at 12 months) and treatment retention than the placebo group.

Sass, Soyka, Mann, and Zieglgansberger (1996) performed a 12-site study in Germany with 272 alcoholic patients. Subjects were administered either 1332 mg of acamprosate for body weight below 60 kg or 1998 mg of acamprosate for body weight above 60 kg or placebo daily. All received counseling or psychotherapy according to customary practice of the participating site. Following 48 weeks of treatment, 43% of acamprosate-treated patients who finished the study had maintained continuous abstinence, versus 25% of placebo-treated subjects. Amazingly, 48 weeks after treatment ceased, 40% of acamprosate-treated patients still remained abstinent, as compared with 17% of the placebo group.

Whitworth et al. (1996) conducted a 1-year, multicenter study of acamprosate in Austria. Four hundred and fifty-five alcohol-dependent patients were randomly administered one of two dose levels of acamprosate as a function of body weight as described above, or placebo daily. At study conclusion, 18% of acamprosate-treated subjects sustained abstinence, versus 7% of placebo-treated patients.

Finally, a 6-month multisite trial of acamprosate was conducted in the Netherlands, Belgium, and Luxembourg, employing 262 alcohol-dependent patients (Geerlings, Ansoms, & van den Brink, 1997). Dosage was adjusted to body weight as described above. Patients treated with acamprosate maintained continuous abstinence longer (45 vs. 15 days), experienced more days abstinent (61 vs. 45 days), and were more likely to be abstinent during the 6 months of treatment (20% vs. 10%) than the placebo-treated group.

Acamprosate is well tolerated and seems to have no serious adverse effects, the most common side effect being diarrhea (Paille et al., 1995; Sass, Soyka, Mann, & Zieglgansberger, 1996; Whitworth et al., 1996). Acamprosate appears to interact with the glutamate receptor (Spanagel & Zieglgansberger, 1997), although its precise mechanism of action is still under investigation.

Disulfiram

Naltrexone and disulfiram (Antabuse) are the only two medications to date approved by the FDA for treatment of alcoholism. Although disulfiram has been available for approximately 50 years, few well-designed studies have been conducted. The most rigorously controlled study was performed by Fuller et al. (1986). In this 1-year, 9-site veteran hospital study, 605 alcohol-dependent patients received either 250 mg of disulfiram per day, 1 mg of disulfiram (placebo) per day, or no disulfiram. No differences were observed among groups in total abstinence, time to first drink, and employment or social stability. However, among subjects who did drink, those who had been on 250 mg of disulfiram drank on fewer days than did those on the 1 mg disulfiram or no disulfiram. Overall, medication compliance was rather low in this study.

Several previous studies have suggested that disulfiram might enhance treatment outcome if compliance-enhancing strategies are employed (Allen & Litten, 1992). Illustrative of this, Chick et al. (1992) conducted a supervised trial in which 200 mg of disulfiram or vitamin C intake was observed daily by an informant. Following 6 months of treatment, patients treated with disulfiram engaged in drinking on fewer days and consumed less alcohol than did the placebo-treated group. In addition, gamma-glutamyl transpeptidase (GGT), a biochemical marker reflecting alcohol consumption, was reduced in disulfiram-treated subjects. In contrast, GGT levels in placebo subjects were elevated.

Finally, recent studies have shown that disulfiram may curb both alcohol and cocaine use in individuals suffering abuse of each substance (Carroll et al., 1993; Higgins, Budney, Bickel, Hughes, & Foerg, 1993). Carroll and colleagues are conducting a rigorous study of disulfiram in this population.

Fluoxetine and Sertraline

Selective serotonin reuptake inhibitors (SSRIs) seem to have potential for treating alcoholics suffering comorbid depression. In the past, only a few well-designed pharmacotherapy trials had been conducted with this population. More recent rigorously controlled studies (Mason, Kocsis, Ritvo, & Cutler, 1996; McGrath et al., 1996) have now shown that the tricyclic antidepressants desipramine and imipramine are helpful in reducing depressive symptoms and likely, to some extent, drinking.

Cornelius et al. (1997) recently completed the first double-blind trial of the SSRI fluoxetine (Prozac) with patients comorbid for alcohol dependence and major depression. Fifty-one patients received between 20 and 40 mg of fluoxetine or placebo daily, as well as standard weekly treatment of supportive psychotherapy and psychiatric sessions. Following 12 weeks of treatment, fluoxetine-treated subjects enjoyed more pronounced improvement in depression than did the placebo group. Furthermore, number of drinking days was significantly reduced by 48% and number of drinks per occasion decreased by 56% in fluoxetine-treated patients. Several well-designed studies are currently underway with the SSRI sertraline (Zoloft) in depressed alcoholics, including a 12-site trial by Pfizer. Brady, Sonne, and Roberts (1995) have also initiated a trial of sertraline with alcoholics evidencing posttraumatic stress disorder.

Future Directions

In spite of recent, important successes in trials of pharmacologic agents, a variety of critical research questions remain unresolved. For example, what is the optimal dose and duration of treatment for naltrexone? What is the physiological basis by which acamprosate diminishes? Would a combination of medications, such as naltrexone and acamprosate, acting on different neuroreceptors of the brain, be more effective than either singly? Since psychosocial interventions are recommended in conjunction with medications, which psychosocial therapy should be used with particular medications and how should the two treatment strategies be integrated? Can specific pharmacologic-psychosocial treatments be matched to different subtypes of alcoholics? Will the medications prove helpful for nondependent, but abusing, patients? Since patient compliance in taking the medication and attending psychotherapy appears to be a key factor in favorable outcome, how can it be fostered? Finally, a host of more fundamental questions surrounding treatment of alcoholics with comorbid psychiatric disorder remain. For instance, how does treatment of either alcoholism or psychiatric disorder affect outcome of the other condition? Also, what sequence of treatment for alcohol and psychiatric problems is optimal?

PHARMACOTHERAPY FOR TREATMENT
OF COCAINE ADDICTION

Over the past decade, extensive research has been conducted on pharmacologic agents to treat cocaine dependency. Unfortunately, no medication has consistently demonstrated efficacy in well-controlled trials. A wide range of drugs has been explored, including stimulants, antidepressants, cocaine antagonists, dopaminergic agents, serotonergic medications, opioid agents, and anticonvulsants (Litten, Allen, Gorelick, & Preston, 1997; Mendelson & Mello, 1996). In spite of the lack of success to date, pharmacotherapy studies continue to address this very serious problem. Experimental agents currently under investigation include desipramine pergolide, a dopamine agonist; risperidone, a dopamine/serotonin antagonist; flupenthixol, a neuroleptic; mazindol, a dopamine reuptake inhibitor; methylphenidate and pemoline, dopamine stimulants; nefazadone, antidepressant and serotonin and norepinephrine reuptake inhibitor and 5-HT$_2$ antagonist; phenytoin, an anticonvulsant; baclofen, a GABAergic agent; amantadine, a dopamine agonist; buprenorphine, a mixed opioid agonist-antagonist; propranolol, a beta-adrenergic antagonist; and memantine, a noncompetive N-methyl-D-aspatate (NMDA) antagonist (Herman, Vocci, Bridge, & Litten, 1996).

Three recent discoveries from basic science may refine the focus of further pharmacotherapy research on cocaine dependence (Leshner, 1996). First, the research team of Giros, Jaber, Jones, Wightman, and Caron (1996) has successfully disabled the gene responsible for transport of dopamine in mice. When administered cocaine, these "knockout" mice did not respond to psychostimulatory effects of cocaine. Volkow et al. (1997) also recently demonstrated an association between the subjective effects of cocaine and blockage of the dopamine transporter in humans. Developing a medication that binds specifically to the dopamine transporter has hence become a high priority.

Second, Self, Barnhart, Lehman, and Nestler (1996) further reinforced the significance of the dopaminergic system in cocaine addiction by showing that activation of D$_1$ and D$_2$ receptors have opposing effects on cocaine-seeking behavior. Future clinical trials will most likely focus on development of medications that interact with dopamine subtype receptors.

Finally, Rocio et al. (1995) employed immunologic techniques to reduce the effects of cocaine. Rats immunized by antibodies against cocaine demonstrated lower psychomotor response and stereotypic behavior in response to cocaine injection. Levels of cocaine were reduced by 52% in the striatal region and 77% in the cerebellum, indicating an antigen-antibody reaction that prevented uptake of cocaine by the brain. Future experiments will no doubt explore use of cocaine antibodies as well as agents that affect pharmacokinetics of cocaine once it is ingested.

PHARMACOTHERAPY FOR OPIATE DEPENDENCE

Methadone, L-alpha-acetylmethadol (LAAM), and naltrexone are currently approved by the FDA to treat opiate dependence. We will briefly review each of these drugs along with a promising new agent, buprenorphine.

Methadone

Methadone, a long-acting opioid agonist and also the most effective pharmacologic maintenance treatment for opiate dependence, acts by reducing acute subjective effects of heroin and other illicit opiates through the mechanism of cross-tolerance. Subsequent reduction in the reinforcement of heroin results in decreased illicit opiate use, crime, and needle sharing (thereby reducing risk of AIDS) and increased treatment retention (Litten, Allen, Gorelick, & Preston, 1997).

In order for methadone treatment to be successful, patients must be clinically managed and monitored appropriately. Maintenance dosing may require 70 mg or more daily (Meandzija & Kosten, 1994). Although there are no serious side effects from long-term use of methadone, minor side effects are common, including constipation, excessive sweating, drowsiness, and decreased sexual interest and performance (Meandzija & Kosten).

LAAM

LAAM, an opioid agonist approved in 1993, differs from methadone on the basis of required frequency of dosing. LAAM is administered every 3 days, while methadone must be given daily. Perhaps the chief disadvantage of LAAM is that a patient may take a considerably longer time to achieve initial stabilization than if given methadone (Herman et al., 1996; Jaffe, 1995). Importantly, LAAM appears as safe as methadone with no serious side effects (Meandzija & Kosten, 1994).

Naltrexone

Naltrexone completely blocks opioid receptors at doses of 50 mg per day. As such, it should be an ideal medication because it blocks the actions of heroin and other opiate agonists. Unfortunately, naltrexone has not proven effective in treatment settings. Treatment retention rates as low as 20% to 30% have been observed after 6 months of treatment (Meandzija & Kosten, 1994). Clearly, poor patient compliance may account for this lack of success (Jaffe, 1995). Low compliance may well be due to the fact that opioid antagonists, unlike methadone and LAAM, do not produce a narcotic effect. In contrast to naltrexone's effect on alcoholics, craving is not reduced in opiate addicts.

Despite this, naltrexone appears useful for individuals highly motivated to quit. Healthcare professionals, business executives, and probationers on naltrexone have been observed to achieve higher success rates than do others (Meandzija & Kosten).

To better ensure patient compliance, the National Institute on Drug Abuse (NIDA) is developing and testing an injectable, long-acting naltrexone, thus eliminating need for daily oral ingestion.

Buprenorphine

Buprenorphine, a "mixed" opioid agonist-antagonist, acting as a partial agonist at the μ opioid receptor and as an antagonist at the kappa opioid receptor (Litten et al., 1997), also seems promising as a means for treating opiate dependence. Several trials have demonstrated its efficacy with opiate-dependent patients (Bickel et al., 1988; Mello & Mendelson, 1980; Mello, Mendelson, & Kuehnle, 1982; Johnson, Jaffe, & Fudala, 1992; Strain, Stitzer, Liebson, & Bigelow, 1994). Buprenorphine reduces heroin use, blocks subjective and physiological effects of other opiates, and augments treatment retention. In addition, it is safe, has little liability of physical dependence, and can be withdrawn or tapered with relative ease (Litten et al.).

Buprenorphine, nevertheless, is subject to abuse. To counteract this, it may be combined with naloxone (Robinson, Dukes, Robinson, Cooke, & Mahoney, 1993). Interestingly, since buprenorphine has a higher affinity than methadone and heroin for μ opioid receptors, addition of naloxone also reduces risk of abuse for these opiates (Litten et al., 1997; Weinhold, Preston, Farre, Liebson, & Bigelow, 1992). NIDA and Reckitt & Colman Pharmaceuticals are collaborating in trials with buprenorphine and buprenorphine/naloxone and opiate-dependent patients in an effort to obtain FDA approval for buprenorphine (Herman et al., 1996).

Future Directions

Since methadone and other opioid agonists and antagonists have not proven totally effective in preventing relapse, research continues on development of medications for opiate dependence. A variety of nonopiate agents have demonstrated promise, including cholecystokinin (CCK) antagonists, serotonergic antianxiety agents, and medications that interact with the glutamate receptor (Herman et al., 1996). In particular, several glutamatergic agents and agents that alter the nitric oxide system have been shown to inhibit mu opioid tolerance (Herman, Vocci, & Bridge, 1995). Among these are noncompetitive and competitive NMDA antagonists, partial glycine agonists, glycine antagonists, and nitric oxide synthase inhibitors. Finally, new proteins related to pain perception are under scientific scrutiny. For example, two new endogenous opiates, endomorphin-1 and endomorphin-2, have recently been isolated (Zadina,

Hackler, Ge, & Kastin, 1997) and may have treatment implications for opiate dependence (Julius, 1997).

PHARMACOTHERAPY FOR NICOTINE DEPENDENCE

In spite of heightened education and prevention strategies, approximately 46 million Americans continue to smoke cigarettes. Nicotine is the most heavily used addictive drug in the United States (NIDA, 1996). Fortunately, nicotine replacement therapy is now readily available to assist these individuals.

Nicotine Replacement

To date, three forms of nicotine replacement products have been approved in the United States: nicotine polacrilex (nicotine gum), transdermally delivered nicotine (nicotine patch), and nasal nicotine spray. The FDA has approved nicotine gum and nicotine patches for purchase over the counter.

Both nicotine gum and the nicotine patch have shown efficacy in heightening short-term abstinence rates, reducing symptoms of nicotine withdrawal, and relieving craving or desire for cigarettes (Hughes; Keenan, Jarvik, & Henningfield, 1994; Rose; Transdermal Nicotine Study Group, 1991). Nicotine replacement therapy, however, is recommended for use with a comprehensive behavioral smoking cessation program (Hughes; Rustin, 1994). Information on clinical use of nicotine gum and patch replacement therapies has been presented by Keenan, Jarvik, and Henningfield (1994) and Rustin (1994).

Nasal nicotine spray, approved by the FDA in the summer of 1996, appears efficacious in sustaining abstinence from smoking (Schneider, Lunell, Olmstead, & Fagerstrom, 1996). An advantage of nasal nicotine spray is that the venous pharmacokinetic profile of nicotine administration closely matches the profile obtained from smoking a cigarette. Other advantages of the spray include simple application and rapid onset of action. Adverse effects include nasal irritation, throat irritation, sneezing, rhinitis, watery eyes, and coughing (Schneider, Lunell, et al., 1996).

The nicotine inhaler is also nearing FDA approval. This device aids in preventing relapse to smoking (Schneider, Olmstead, et al., 1996). Common side effects, however, are throat and mouth irritation and coughing.

Bupropion

Bupropion (Zyban), a medication approved to treat depression (under the trade name Wellbutrin), was approved by the FDA in May 1997 as an aid to smoking cessation treatment.

In a recent study by Hurt, Glover, Sachs, Dale, and Schroeder (1996) a dose-response study of bupropion was conducted in 615 smokers. Subjects received either 100 mg, 150 mg, or 300 mg of a sustained-release (SR) form of bupropion or placebo daily. After 7 weeks of active treatment, patients were followed for 1 year. Smoking cessation rates of the 150 mg and 300 mg groups at the end of treatment and at the end of the 1-year posttreatment significantly exceeded those of the placebo group. In addition, bupropion was well tolerated.

Most recently, a trial was conducted contrasting bupropion, nicotine, and bupropion and nicotine in combination (Glaxo Wellcome, 1997). Eight hundred and ninety-three chronic smokers were administered either 300 mg of bupropion SR, 21 mg of nicotine from a nicotine patch (Habitrol); combined 300 mg of bupropion SR plus 21 mg of nicotine from a nicotine patch, or placebo daily. Patients also received individual smoking cessation and relapse prevention therapy. Following 7 weeks of treatment, abstinence rates during weeks 4 through 7 were 23% for subjects receiving placebo, 36% for nicotine patch, 49% for bupropion, and 58% for combined bupropion and nicotine. The trial is ongoing.

Although bupropion is contraindicated in patients with a seizure disorder, overall it appears quite safe. The most common side effects are dry mouth and insomnia (Glaxo Wellcome, 1997). Bupropion's mechanism of action remains unknown. It is a weak blocker of the neuronal uptake of serotonin, norepinephrine, and dopamine, the latter believed to be involved in the positive reinforcement for smoking (Dani & Heinemann, 1996).

Future Directions

A possible alternative to agonist (nicotine) replacement therapy is blockage of the nicotine receptor. For example, the nicotine antagonist acamylamine increases abstinence rates in smoking when used in conjunction with a nicotine patch (Rose et al., 1994).

Investigators are also exploring reward neuropathways stimulated by smoking and comparing their activity with that underlying the positive reinforcement produced by alcohol and other drugs of abuse. For example, it is possible that other neurotransmitter systems, such as the mesolimbic dopamine system, implicated in the reinforcement of cocaine and opioid abuse, may play a role in smoking behavior (Dani & Heinemann, 1996). Research on pharmacologic agents that alter these neurotransmitter systems may lead to agents to prevent or reduce smoking, particularly if the medication is used in combination with nicotine replacement therapy. Bupropion represents a successful employment of this strategy.

Finally, a high proportion of individuals dependent on alcohol and other drugs are also nicotine dependent. It is important to explore how the treatment of alcoholism and other addictive drugs may contribute to reduction of nicotine dependence.

CONCLUSION

As discussed earlier, a wide range of medicational adjuncts are now available or will likely soon be available to assist in the treatment of substance-dependence disorders. Other promising medications are in earlier stages of development and require more extensive research. It is important to determine how these agents can be employed to best avail. While several have demonstrated efficacy, none should be viewed as a "magic bullet." Future research is likely to extend to exploration of medications in combination with each other as well as in combination with effective psychosocial interventions. The National Institute on Alcohol Abuse and Alcoholism has recently initiated a multisite clinical trial that will evaluate two promising drugs separately and in combination, as well as consider how the agents may augment efficacy of two intensities of behavioral treatment for alcoholism (Schneider, Olmstead, et al., 1996).

REFERENCES

Allen, J. P., & Litten, R. Z. (1992). Techniques to enhance compliance with disulfiram. *Alcoholism, Clinical and Experimental Research, 16*, 1035–1041.

Bickel, W. K., Stitzer, M. L., Bigelow, G. W., Liebson, K. A., Jasinski, D. R., & Johnson, R. E. (1988). A clinical trial of buprenorphine: Comparison with methadone in the detoxification of heroin addicts. *Clinical Pharmacology and Therapeutics, 43*, 72–78.

Brady, K. T., Sonne, S. C., & Roberts, J. M. (1995). Sertraline treatment of comorbid posttraumatic stress disorder and alcohol dependence. *Journal of Clinical Psychiatry, 56*, 502–505.

Carroll, K., Ziedonis, D., O'Malley, S., McCance-Katz, E., Gordon, L., & Rounsaville, B. (1993). Pharmacologic interventions for alcohol- and cocaine-abusing individuals. *The American Journal on Addictions, 2*, 77–79.

Chick, J., Gough, K., Falkowski, W., Kershaw, P., Hore, B., Mehta, B., Ritson, B., Ropner, R., & Torley, D. (1992). Disulfiram treatment of alcoholism. *British Journal of Psychiatry, 161*, 84–89.

Cornelius, J. R., Salloum, I. M., Ehler, J. G., Jarrett, P. J., Cornelius, M. D., Perel, J. M., Thase, M. E., & Black, A. (1997). Fluoxetine in depressed alcoholics: A double-line placebo-controlled trial. *Archives of General Psychiatry, 54*, 700–705.

Croop, R. S., Faulkner, E. B., & Labriola, D. F. (1997). The safety profile of naltrexone in the treatment of alcoholism. *Archives of General Psychiatry, 54*, 1130–1135.

Dani, J. A., & Heinemann, S. (1996). Molecular and cellular aspects of nicotine abuse. *Neuron, 16*, 905–908.

Fuller, R. K., Branchey, L., Brightwell, D. R., Derman, R. M., Emrick, C. D., Iber, F. L., James, K. E., Lacourseire, R. B., Lee, K. K., Lowstam, I., Maany, I., Neiderhiser, D., Nocks, J. J., & Shaw, S. (1986). Disulfiram treatment of alcoholism: A Veterans Administration cooperative study. *Journal of the American Medical Association, 256*, 1449–1455.

Geerlings, P. J., Ansoms, C., & van den Brink, W. (1997). Acamprosate and prevention of relapse in alcoholics. *European Addiction Research 3*, 129–137.

Gerra, G., Caccavari, R., Delsignore, R., Bocchi, R., Fertonani, G., & Passeri, M., 1992. Effects of fluoxetine and Ca-acetyl-homotaurine on alcohol intake in familial and nonfamilial alcoholics patients. *Current Therapeutic Research, 52*, 291–295.

Giros, B., Jaber, M., Jones, S. R., Wightman, R. M., & Caron, M. G. (1996). Hyperlocomotion and indifference to cocaine and amphetamine in mice lacking the dopamine transporter. *Nature, 379,* 606–612.

Glaxo Wellcome. (1997). *Use of bupropion hydrochloride in smoking cessation therapy.* Research Triangle Park, NC: Author.

Herman, B. H., Vocci, F., & Bridge, P. (1995). The effects of NMDA receptor antagonists and nitric oxide synthase inhibitors on opioid tolerance and withdrawal: Medication development issues for opiate addiction. *Neuropsychopharmacology, 13,* 269–293.

Herman, B. H., Vocci, F., Bridge, P., & Litten, R. Z. (1996). *Medications development for opiate, cocaine, and alcohol dependence.* Paper presented for American Academy of Child and Adolescent Psychiatry, Philadelphia.

Higgins, S. T., Budney, A. J., Bickel, W. K., Hughes, J. R., & Foerg, F. (1993). Disulfiram therapy in patients abusing cocaine and alcohol. *American Journal of Psychiatry, 150,* 675–676.

Hughes, J. R., Gust, S. W., Keenan, R. M., Fenwick, J. W., & Healey, M. L. (1989). Nicotine vs placebo gum in general medical practice. *Journal of American Medical Association, 261,* 1300–1305.

Hughes, J. R., Gust, S. W., Keenan, R., Fenwick, J. W., Skoog, K., & Higgins, S. T. (1991). Long-term use of nicotine vs placebo gum. *Archives of Internal Medicine, 151,* 1991–1998.

Hurt, R. D., Glover, E. D., Sachs, D. P. L., Dale, L. C., & Schroeder, D. R. (1996). Bupropion for smoking cessation: A double-blind, placebo-controlled dose response trial. *Journal of Addictive Diseases, 15,* 137.

Jaffe, J. H. (1995). Pharmacological treatment of opioid dependence: Current techniques and new findings. *Psychiatric Annals, 25,* 369–375.

Julius, D., 1997. Another opiate for the masses? *Nature 386,* 442.

Johnson, R. E., Jaffe, J. H., & Fudala, P. J. (1992). A controlled trial of buprenorphine treatment for opioid dependence. *Journal of the American Medical Association, 267,* 2750–2755.

Keenan, R. M., Jarvik, M. E., & Henningfield, J. E. (1994). Management of nicotine dependence and withdrawal. In N. A. Miller (Ed.), *Principles of addiction medicine* (pp. 1–11, Section XI, Chapter 7). Chevy Chase, MD: American Society of Addiction Medicine.

Leshner, A. I. (1996). Molecular mechanisms of cocaine. *The New England Journal of Medicine, 335,* 128–129.

Lhuintre, J. P., Daoust, M., Moore, N. D., Chretien, P., Saligaut, C., Tran, G., Boismare, F., & Hillemand, B. (1985). Ability of calcium acetyl homotaurine, a GABA agonist, to prevent relapse in weaned alcoholics. *The Lancet, 1,* 1014–1016.

Lhuintre, J. P., Moore, N., Tran, G., Steru, L., Langrenon, S., Daoust, M., Parot, Ph., Ladure, Ph., Libert, C., Boismare, F., & Hillemand, B. (1990). Acamprosate appears to decrease alcohol intake in weaned alcoholics. *Alcohol and Alcoholism, 25,* 613–622.

Litten, R. Z., Allen, J. P., Gorelick, D. A., & Preston, K. (1997). Experimental pharmacological agents to reduce alcohol, cocaine, and opiate use. In N. S. Miller (Ed.), *The principles and practice of addictions in psychiatry* (pp. 532–567). Philadelphia, PA: W.B. Saunders.

Litten, R. Z., & Fertig, J. (1996, November). International update: New findings on promising medications. *Alcoholism, Clinical and Experimental Research,* suppl., 216A–218A.

Mann, K., Chabac, S., Lehert, P., Potgieter, A., & Sass, H. (1995). *Acamprosate improves treatment outcome in alcoholics: A polled analysis of 11 randomized placebo con-*

trolled trials in 3338 patients. Poster presented at the Annual Conference of the American College of Neuropsychopharmacology, Puerto Rico.

Mason, B. J., Kocsis, J. H., Ritvo, E. C., & Cutler, R. B. (1996). A double-blind placebo-controlled trial of desipramine in primary alcoholics stratified on the presence or absence of major depression. *Journal of the American Medical Association, 275*, 1–7.

McGrath, P. J., Nunes, E. V., Stewart, J. W., Goldman, D., Agosti, V., Ocepek-Welikson, K., & Quitkin, F. M. (1996). Imipramine treatment of alcoholics with primary depression: A placebo-controlled clinical trial. *Archives of General Psychiatry, 53*, 232–240.

Meandzija, B., & Kosten, T. R. (1994). Pharmacologic therapies for opioid addiction. In N.S. Miller (Ed.), *Principles of addiction medicine* (pp. 1–5 Section XII, Chapter 4). Chevy Chase, MD: American Society of Addiction Medicine.

Mello, N. K., & Mendelson, J. H. (1980). Buprenorphine suppresses heroin use by heroin addicts. *Science, 207*, 657–659.

Mello, N. K., Mendelson, J. H., & Kuehnle, J. C. (1982). Buprenorphine effects on human heroin self-administration: An operant analysis. *The Journal of Pharmacology and Experimental Therapeutics, 223*, 30–39.

Mendelson, J. H., & Mello, N. K. (1996). Management of cocaine abuse and dependence. *The New England Journal of Medicine, 334*, 965–972.

National Institute on Drug Abuse. (1996). Cigarette smoking. In *NIDA Capsules* (Report No. C-83-08, January Issue). Rockville, MD: Press Office of the National Institute on Drug Abuse.

O'Brien, C. P., & McLellan, A. T. (1996). Myths about the treatment of addiction. *The Lancet, 347*, 237–240.

O'Malley, S. S., Jaffe, A. J., Chang, G., Schottenfield, R. S., Meyer, R. E., & Rounsaville, B. (1992). Naltrexone and coping skills therapy for alcohol dependence: A controlled study. *Archives of General Psychiatry, 49*, 881–887.

Paille, F. M., Guelfi, J. D., Perkins, A. C., Royer, R. J., Steru, L., & Parot, P. (1995). Double-blind randomized multicentre trial of acamprosate in maintaining abstinence from alcohol. *Alcohol and Alcoholism, 30*, 239–247.

Robinson, G. M., Dukes, P. D., Robinson, B. J., Cooke, R. R., & Mahoney, G. N. (1993). The misuse of buprenorphine and a buprenorphine-naloxone combination in Wellington, New Zealand. *Drug and Alcohol Dependence, 33*, 81–86.

Rocio, M., Carrera, A., Ashley, J. A., Parsons, L. H., Wirsching, P., Koob, G. F., & Janda, K. D. (1995). Suppression of psychoactive effects of cocaine by active immunization. *Nature, 378*, 727–730.

Rose, J. E., Behm, F. M., Westman, E. C., Levin, E. D., Stein, R. M., & Ripka, G. V. (1994). Mecamylamine combined with nicotine skin patch facilitates smoking cessation beyond nicotine patch treatment alone. *Clinical Pharmacology and Therapeutics, 56*, 86–99.

Rose, J. E., Levin, E. D., Behm, F. M., Adivi, C., & Schur, C. (1990). Transdermal nicotine facilitates smoking cessation. *Clinical Pharmacology and Therapeutics, 47*, 323–330.

Rustin, T. A. (1994). Pharmacologic therapies for nicotine addiction. In N. S. Miller (Ed.), *Principles of addiction medicine* (pp. 1–8, Section XII, Chapter 5). Chevy Chase, MD: American Society of Addiction Medicine.

Sass, H., Soyka, M., Mann, K., & Zieglgansberger, W. (1996). Relapse prevention by acamprosate: Results from a placebo-controlled study on alcohol dependence. *Archives of General Psychiatry, 53*, 673–680.

Schneider, N. G., Lunell, E., Olmstead, R. E., & Fagerstrom, K. O. (1996). Clinical pharmacokinetics of nasal nicotine delivery: A review and comparison to other nicotine systems. *Clinical Pharmacokinetics, 31*, 65–80.

Schneider, N. G., Olmstead, R., Nisson, F., Mody, F. V., Franzon, M., & Doan, K. (1996). Efficacy of a nicotine inhaler in smoking cessation: A double-blind, placebo-controlled trial. *Addiction, 91,* 1293–1306.

Self, D. W., Barnhart, W. J., Lehman, D. A., & Nestler, E. J. (1996). Opposite modulation of cocaine-seeking behavior by D_1- and D_2-like dopamine receptor agonists. *Science, 271,* 1586–1589.

Spanagel, R., & Zieglgansberger, W. (1997). Anti-craving compounds for ethanol: New pharmacological tools to study addictive processes. *Trends in Pharmacological Sciences, 18,* 54–59.

Strain, E. C., Stitzer, M. L., Liebson, I. A., & Bigelow, G. E. (1994). Comparison of buprenorphine and methadone in the treatment of opioid dependence. *American Journal of Psychiatry, 151,* 1025–1030.

Transdermal Nicotine Study Group. (1991). Transdermal nicotine for smoking cessation: Six-month results from two multicenter controlled clinical trials. *Journal of the American Medical Association, 266,* 3133–3138.

Volkow, N. D., Wang, G. J., Fischman, M. W., Foltin, R. W., Fowler, J. S., Abumrad, N. N., Vitkun, S., Logan, J., Gatlery, S. J., Pappas, N., Hitzemann, R., & Shea, C. E. (1997). Relationship between subjective effects of cocaine and dopamine transporter occupancy. *Nature, 386,* 827–830.

Volpicelli, J. R., Alterman, A. I., Hayashida, M., & O'Brien, C. P. (1992). Naltrexone in the treatment of alcohol dependence. *Archives of General Psychiatry, 49,* 876–880.

Volpicelli, J. R., Rhines, K. C., Rhines, J. S., Volpicelli, L. A., Alterman, A. I., & O'Brien, C. P. (1997). Naltrexone and alcohol dependence: Role of subject compliance. *Archives of General Psychiatry, 54,* 737–742.

Weinhold, L. L., Preston, K. L., Farre, M., Liebson, I. A., & Bigelow, G. E. (1992). Buprenorphine alone and in combination with naloxone in non-dependent humans. *Drug and Alcohol Dependence, 30,* 263–274.

Whitworth, A. B., Fischer, F., Lesch, O. M., Nimmerrichter, A., Oberbauer, H., Platz, T., Potgieter, A., Walter, H., & Fleischhacker, W. W. (1996). Comparison of acamprosate and placebo in long-term treatment of alcohol dependence. *The Lancet, 347,* 1438–1442.

Zadina, J. E., Hackler, L., Ge, L. J., & Kastin, A. J. (1997). A potent and selective endogenous agonist for the μ-opiate receptor. *Nature, 386,* 499–502.

Chapter 2

The Pharmacotherapy of Relapse Prevention Using Anticonvulsants

Thomas R. Kosten, M.D.

In this chapter we review the preclinical rationale for using anticonvulsants to prevent relapse in substance abusers. The major group of substance abusers who have been studied are stimulant-dependent patients, although anticonvulsants clearly have a role in the detoxification of patients from sedating agents, such as alcohol, as reviewed in the previous chapters in this book. Because the preclinical rationale for using anticonvulsants to prevent relapse is dependent on the concept of craving, anticonvulsants may be more broadly useful for all substances that are associated with craving. A critical assumption in this generalization, however, is that craving is similar across various drugs of abuse. But this assumption may not be accurate. The craving associated with drugs that produce significant withdrawal appears to be different from the craving associated with drugs that primarily have euphoria as their driving motivation for use. After reviewing the existing clinical trials using anticonvulsants to prevent relapse in stimulant abusers, we will consider whether a specific comorbid subgroup of patients may specifically benefit from anticonvulsant treatment for relapse prevention. Because anticonvulsants have demonstrated efficacy in the treatment of bipolar disorders, those patients with both substance abuse and bipolar disorder might particularly benefit from anticonvulsant treatment.

The rationale for using anticonvulsants for relapse prevention in the treatment of substance abuse is based on a hypothesized connection between kindling and drug craving (Halikas & Kuhn, 1990). The kindling phenomenon

This study was supported by National Institute on Drug Abuse Grants P50 DA09250 and P50 DA04060.

involves a progressive facilitation of neuronal firing leading to a lowered seizure threshold after repeated stimulation with seizure-inducing agents, such as stimulants (Goddard, McIntyre, & Leech, 1969; Post, Ballenger, et al., 1981; Post & Kopanda, 1975, 1976; Post, Kopanda, & Black, 1976; Tatum & Seevers, 1929). Agents do not need to be given at dosages that actually would produce seizures during these kindling-inducing sessions. Due to sensitization, the amount of stimulant that is needed to induce a seizure becomes smaller and smaller after repeated administration of stimulants. For example, repeated administration of cocaine at relatively large but non-seizure-inducing dosages will eventually lead to the induction of seizures in animals at dosages that would not initially have induced seizures. Sensitization contrasts to tolerance, which is associated with less and less effect as a drug is repeatedly given. The stimulant administration parameters contributing to sensitization rather than tolerance are complex but involve relatively large dosages of the substance given at relatively widely spaced intervals compared with the drug's half-life (Post & Kopanda, 1975). Tolerance induction usually involves more modest but often escalating dosages of a drug given in relatively rapid sequences compared with the half-life of the drug. Because of the patterns of stimulant use by humans, both tolerance during acute binges of usage and sensitization over prolonged periods of years or months of usage might be expected to develop (Gawin & Ellinwood, 1988).

In 1992, Halikas et al. published a pilot study using carbamazepine in 35 outpatients with self-reported cocaine use as the outcome measure. They categorized these patients into three groups: those with a marked decrease in use, those with a more modest decrease in cocaine use, and those with no change. Thirteen patients reported a marked decrease in use, going from 65 days of use per 100 days to 3 days of use per 100 days during a several-month trial. The second group of 13 with more modest reduction in use went from 78 days of use per 100 days to 35 days of use per 100 days. Finally, the third group of 9 subjects showed no change and in fact refused to continue on the medications during this pilot study.

In this pilot study, compliance with the medication was a critical determinant of treatment outcome. The target medication dose was 600 mg daily of carbamazepine, and the average dose ingested was 350 mg per day. Compliance was correlated with both reduced drug use and reduced craving. Using a 100-point scale to assess cocaine craving, those patients with zero days of compliance per week averaged 58 on this scale, those patients with 1–2 days of compliance per week averaged 50, those with 3–5 days averaged 37, and those with 6–7 days of compliance per week averaged a score of 40. This produced a highly significant correlation between days of compliance per week and reported cocaine craving scores. A similar association was shown between self-reported cocaine use and compliance. Those subjects with more than 75% compliance with daily carbamazepine use showed a 66% reduction in cocaine use, whereas those showing between 25% and 75% compliance showed only a

50% reduction in cocaine use. While the authors ascribed some of the success to the medication itself, a causal association could as easily be drawn between compliance with treatment in general and reduction in cocaine use. The one clear association between compliance and carbamazepine effects was found in methadone-maintained patients, where carbamazepine compliance was clearly associated with the precipitation of opiate withdrawal symptoms.

The next study by Halikas and his group (1991) was a double-blind placebo-controlled crossover study with 32 crack cocaine abusers. In this 20-day study, patients were crossed over between placebo and carbamazepine at either 200 mg or 400 mg daily. Using urine toxicologies as the outcome measure, less cocaine use was noted during carbamazepine treatment than during placebo. During carbamazepine treatment, only 22% of the urines were positive for cocaine metabolites. Again, some association appeared to occur between compliance and reductions in cocaine use because subjects with carbamazepine levels above 4 μ/ml had a better outcome than those having lower blood levels. These blood levels were not well correlated with the two different dosages of carbamazepine.

Based on these initial positive findings, three larger scale placebo-controlled parallel-group randomized clinical trials were undertaken. The study by Cornish et al. (1995) enrolled 82 subjects and monitored blood levels of carbamazepine in order to have a target between 4 and 12 μ/ml. In this 10-week trial with outpatients, they had 55% retention with no significant difference between the placebo and medicated group, although the carbamazepine group had somewhat higher retention during weeks 1 to 4. The percentage of cocaine-positive urines showed no difference between the placebo and medication groups (36% vs. 25%).

A similar study by Kranzler et al. (1995) enrolled 40 subjects in a placebo-controlled trial. In this 12-week study, the medicated group received 600 mg/day of carbamazepine and showed a good retention rate of 60% with no difference between the placebo and medicated group. Urine toxicologies also showed no difference between the two groups (66% vs. 76% positive for cocaine metabolites). An interesting finding in this study occurred at a 3-month follow-up after the medication had been discontinued. Those subjects who had been treated with carbamazepine reported less alcohol use than those patients who had been treated with placebo (3.6 vs. 8.1 days of drinking per month). Since this difference was not evident at the end of the medication treatment phase, it is somewhat difficult to ascribe this to carbamazepine effects. Instead, these anticonvulsants may have some role in the more extended treatment of alcoholic patients beyond the initial detoxification phase, where anticonvulsants have demonstrated efficacy.

The third randomized clinical trial by Montoya et al. (1995) involved 62 subjects in a somewhat more complex design. Subjects were enrolled in an 8-week trial in which they received escalating and then decreasing dosages of carbamazepine. The peak dose was 800 mg/day, which occurred at the middle week of this trial. Subjects were treated with lower dosages in the weeks leading up to Week 4 and in the weeks after this dosage. A comparison group received placebos throughout the 8 weeks. Retention in this trial was somewhat lower than in the previous trials, but interestingly, the carbamazepine group had somewhat higher retention than the placebo group during Weeks 3 to 5. Cocaine use did not differ between the placebo and carbamazepine group, and in contrast to the previous studies, there was no significant change in cocaine use for either group compared with baseline.

The most recent study using carbamazepine in cocaine abusers was published by Halikas et al. (1997) and involved a 12-week double-blind study that compared placebo to carbamazepine at 400 and 800 mg/day. The initial randomization included 183 subjects, of whom 57 completed this 12-week study. Ninety percent compliance with the medication was reported, and retention in the trial was correlated with blood levels of carbamazepine as categorized from 0 to 4, 6, and 8 μ/ml blood level. This retention difference was particularly evident from Weeks 5 through 8. At Weeks 5 and 6, the retention was 95% in the 15 subjects with blood levels greater than 8 μ/ml, whereas the placebo group at this time period had only 60% retention. Beyond Week 8, there appeared to be no difference in retention based on blood levels or placebo vs. medicated groups. Urine toxicologies were analyzed using hierarchical linear modeling and no difference was found between the 800 μ/day group and placebo, although the 400 mg/day group appeared to show a significant reduction in positive cocaine urines compared with either of the other two groups. Once again, blood levels of carbamazepine were significantly related to lower levels of cocaine-positive urines. Thus compliance again appears to be the most important factor in determining success using this medication. Despite their statistical significance, the clinical significance in the rates of cocaine-positive urines appeared to be fairly minimal. In the 400 mg/day group, the baseline rate of cocaine urines was 63%; during the trial this rate dropped to 47%, and at the last visit the rate was down to 41% cocaine-positive urines. For the placebo group, the rate was 64% at baseline, 53% during the trial, and 55% at the last visit. For the 800 mg/day group, the rate was 49% at baseline, 49% during the trial, and 57% at the last visit. Thus the reduction of about 20% in cocaine-positive urines for the 400 mg/day group was not that different from the reduction of about 10% for the placebo group.

In summary, the role of carbamazepine and perhaps other anticonvulsants in stimulant abuse treatment appears to be limited based on the controlled clinical trials. Further, the theoretical rationale for this use may need reexamination. Intermittent stimulant administration leading to sensitization augments certain effects, such as motor hyperactivity and seizures in rodent models, but the role for such sensitization in humans is less clear (Chaudhry, Turkanis, & Karler, 1988; Tatum & Seevers, 1929). Sensitization has been suggested as an important part of the paranoia and panic attacks seen in stimulant abusers, but the relationship of sensitization to craving has been described in only a single case report (Halikas & Kuhn, 1990; Jones, 1985). This case suggested a kindling phenomenon, but a temporal correspondence between the craving reports and kindling was not evident. Furthermore, craving as a precipitant of relapse is not firmly established: Instead of being a precipitant for the initial cocaine use of a relapse, craving may be a result of that use. Craving is frequently intensified by even modest cocaine use (Kosten et al., 1992). Another limitation in the kindling model for humans is that humans rarely use stimulants on a schedule that has been shown in animal models to facilitate kindling. However, if the lower dosages used by humans did induce kindling, then this phenomenon should be much more widespread among any users of cocaine. Since only 10% of users progress on to dependence and severe abuse, the importance of kindling as a component of relapse or even progression to dependence seems minimal. Other data questioning the importance of kindling are that many other medications can produce kindling but have no abuse potential (Post et al., 1981). The relationship of kindling to craving is further brought into question by the persistence of kindling after its induction in animal models. In contrast, a relatively rapid reduction in craving can be seen within a week or two of entering treatment (Kosten, 1992; O'Brien et al., 1988). Thus the conceptual model linking kindling to craving and to relapse in humans appears relatively weak and needs reconsideration.

The treatment strategy of using anticonvulsants or carbamazepine specifically is similarly problematic. Carbamazepine is useful for preventing the development of sensitization and kindling but not for its reversal once sensitization is established (Post, 1988; Post & Kopanda, 1975). Thus carbamazepine would appear to have more of a role in patients who are early career users of cocaine or who are already abstinent from stimulants for relatively longer periods of time and have had some opportunity to work on relapse prevention. Because carbamazepine may prevent the development of further sensitization or kindling, relapse prevention in early career users may be a future role for carbamazepine treatment.

Three possible areas are suggested for future research. First, patients with higher serum levels of carbamazepine appeared to have better early retention. This was found by Cornish et al. (1995), Halikas et al. (1997), and Montoya et al. (1995). These higher serum levels are of course confounded by better compliance, which will lead to higher blood levels, and patients with better compliance to treatment are more likely to remain in treatment. Overall, the changes in urine toxicologies have been quite modest or nonexistent in these controlled studies. Second, there may be a possible delayed response in alcoholic/cocaine users (Kranzler et al., 1995). Whether this suggests the extended use of carbamazepine beyond detoxification in alcoholic patients is an interesting question worthy of future studies. The recent long-term (12-month) placebo-controlled study by Mueller et al. (1997) in 29 alcoholics found that despite compliance problems beyond 4 months and sizable dropout, the carbamazepine group showed a significant decrease in drinks per drinking day and maximum number of heavy drinking days in a row at 2 and 4 months. There was also a significant delay in time to first heavy drinking episode (15% vs. 45% at 3 months). Third, there may be a good response in patients with bipolar or perhaps more generally affective disorders. This hypothesis is worth continued study with trials focusing on this particular subgroup.

REFERENCES

Chaudhry, I. A., Turkanis, S. A., & Karler, R. (1988). Characteristics of reverse tolerance to amphetamine-induced locomotor stimulation in mice. *Neuropharmacology, 27,* 777–781.

Cornish, J. W., Maany, I., Fudala, P. J., et al. (1995). Carbamazepine treatment for cocaine dependence. *Drug and Alcohol Dependence, 38,* 221–227.

Gawin, F., & Ellinwood, E. H. (1992). Cocaine and other stimulants. *New England Journal of Medicine, 318,* 1173–1182.

Goddard, G. V., McIntyre, D. C., & Leech, C. K. (1969). A permanent change in brain functioning resulting from daily electrical stimulation. *Experimental Neurology, 25,* 295.

Halikas, J. A., Crosby, R. D., Carlson, G. A., et al. (1991). Cocaine reduction in unmotivated crack users using carbamazepine versus placebo in a short-term cross-over design. *Clinical Pharmacology and Therapeutics, 50,* 81–95.

Halikas, J. A., Crosby, R. D., Pearson, V. L., et al. (1997). A randomized double-blind study of carbamazepine in the treatment of cocaine abuse. *Clinical Pharmacology and Therapeutics, 62,* 89–105.

Halikas, J. A., & Kuhn, K. L. (1990). A possible neurophysiological basis of cocaine craving. *Annals of Clinical Psychiatry, 2,* 79–83.

Halikas, J. A., Kuhn, K. L., Carlson, G. A., et al. (1992). The effect of carbamazepine on cocaine use. *The American Journal on Addictions, 1,* 30–39.

Jones, R. (1985). The pharmacology of cocaine. In J. Grabowski (Ed.), *Cocaine: Pharmacology, effects, and treatment of abuse: Vol. 50: NIDA Research Monographs* (pp. 34–48). Rockville, MD: National Institute on Drug Abuse.

Kosten, T. R. (1992). Can cocaine craving be a medication development outcome? Drug craving and relapse in opioid and cocaine dependence. *The American Journal on Addictions, 1,* 230–239.

Kosten, T. R., Gawin, F. H., Silverman, D. G., et al. (1992). Intravenous cocaine challenges during desipramine maintenance. *Neuropsychopharmacology, 7,* 169–176.

Kranzler, H. R., Bauer, L. O., Hersh, D., et al. (1995). Carbamazepine treatment of cocaine dependence: A placebo-controlled trial. *Drug and Alcohol Dependence, 38,* 203–211.

Montoya, I. D., Levin, F. R., Fudala, P. J., et al. (1995). Double-blind comparison of carbamazepine and placebo for treatment of cocaine dependence. *Drug and Alcohol Dependence, 38,* 213–219.

Mueller, T. I., Stout, R. L., Rudden, S., et al. (1997). A double-blind, placebo-controlled pilot study of carbamazepine for the treatment of alcohol dependence. *Alcoholism, Clinical and Experimental Research, 21,* 86–92.

O'Brien, C., Childress, A. R., Arndt, I., et al. (1988). Pharmacological and behavioral treatments of cocaine dependence: Controlled studies. *Journal of Clinical Psychiatry, 49,* 17–23.

Post, R. M. (1988). Time course of clinical effects of carbamazepine: Implications for mechanism of action. *Journal of Clinical Psychiatry, 49* (suppl. 1), 35–36.

Post, R. M., Ballenger, J. C., Uhde, T. W., et al. (1981). Kindling and drug sensitization: Implications for the progressive development of psychopathology and treatment with carbamazepine. In M. Sandler (Ed.), *The psychopharmacology of anti-convulsants* (pp. 29–48). Oxford, UK: Oxford University Press.

Post, R. M., & Kopanda, R. T. (1976). Cocaine, kindling and psychosis. *American Journal of Psychiatry, 133,* 627–634.

Post, R. M., & Kopanda, R. T. (1975). Cocaine, kindling and reverse tolerance. *Lancet, 1*(7903), 409–410.

Post, R. M., Kopanda, R. T., & Black, K. E. (1976). Progressive effects of cocaine on behavior and central amine metabolism in rhesus monkeys: Relationships to kindling and psychosis. *Biological Psychiatry, 11,* 403–419.

Tatum, A. L., & Seevers, M. H. (1929). Experimental cocaine addiction. *Journal of Pharmacology and Experimental Therapy, 36,* 401–410.

Chapter 3

Current Developments
in Psychosocial Treatments
of Alcohol and Substance Abuse

Lynne Siqueland, Ph.D.
Paul Crits-Christoph, Ph.D.

INTRODUCTION

Drug abuse and dependence remains a significant problem in the United States. The latest NIDA Household Survey (1996) completed in 1996 reports that an estimated 13 million Americans had used an illicit drug during the past month. Clinical and prison populations, as well as the homeless, have higher prevalences of both substance use disorders and dual diagnoses with mental illness (Regier et al., 1990). Although there have been some exciting developments in medications that help in treating alcohol abuse (e.g., naltrexone), and methadone aids the treatment of opiate addiction, there is still no definitive medication treatment for marijuana or cocaine dependence. Even with the medications as adjuncts, psychosocial interventions and self-help programs have formed the backbone of substance abuse treatment. In this article, we review recent developments and promising interventions from both clinical trials and naturalistic studies that have appeared in the past year for the treatment of alcohol, cocaine, and opiate abuse or dependence.

RANDOMIZED CLINICAL TRIALS

Alcohol

A number of articles from the Project MATCH Research Group in 1998 continue to provide information about whether it is possible to match patients to treatment based on pretreatment patient characteristics. In 1997, Project MATCH published their first major outcome paper looking at the treatment outcomes at 1-year follow-up. In 1998, they separately published findings about the end of active-phase (12 weeks) treatment (Project MATCH, 1998b)[1] and 3-year follow-up outcomes (Project MATCH, 1998a).[2] Project MATCH compared 12-step facilitation therapy (TSF), cognitive-behavioral therapy (CBT), and motivational enhancement therapy (MET) with both an outpatient and aftercare sample of over 1,500 alcoholic patients (Project MATCH, 1997). CBT was based in social learning principles and focused on overcoming skill deficits and teaching patients to cope with triggers or situations (intrapsychic and interpersonal) associated with relapse. TSF was focused on helping the patient incorporate the belief system of Alcoholics Anonymous (AA), become an active participant in AA, and work on the first three recovery steps of AA. MET, based on motivational psychology and the natural recovery process, focused on the individual's own coping resources and identified those resources available in the patient's community. TSF and CBT were 12 sessions in length with once-a-week sessions, whereas MET included a total of 4 sessions. The goal of Project MATCH was to compare drinking outcome in the three treatments and, more importantly, to attempt to identify factors on which patients could be matched to particular treatments. Matching variables included psychiatric severity, severity of alcohol use, social support for drinking, readiness to change, meaning seeking, sociopathy, typology, cognitive impairment, client conceptual level, and gender.

Project MATCH (1998b) reported that TSF and CBT had better outcome at posttreatment on alcohol consumption and alcohol-related negative consequences than MET, but TSF and CBT did not differ from each other. These results were only true for the outpatient sample. Of the patients in TSF and CBT, 41% were abstinent or drinking moderately without alcohol-related consequences compared with 28% of the MET patients (Figure 3.1). There were no differences among the three treatments on measures of employment, psychologic or social functioning, or liver functioning. None of the matching variables had any effect on outcome at 12 weeks.

Despite this interesting result of differences between the treatments at the end of 12 weeks, these differences were not maintained at the 1-year follow-up (Project MATCH, 1997). The study authors suggest that treatment in-

---

1. Project MATCH found that 12-step facilitation therapy (TSF) and cognitive-behavioral therapy (CBT) had better outcomes immediately posttreatment on alcohol consumption and alcohol-related negative consequences than motivational enhancement therapy (MET) in an outpatient sample of over 700 alcoholic patients. None of the patient–treatment matching hypotheses were confirmed.

2. This paper reports on the 3-year outcome for the Project MATCH (1998a) study described above. Treatment gains found at 1 year were maintained at 3 years with a slight advantage for TSF on a total abstinence measure. The patient–treatment matching variables of anger and networks supportive of drinking are discussed.

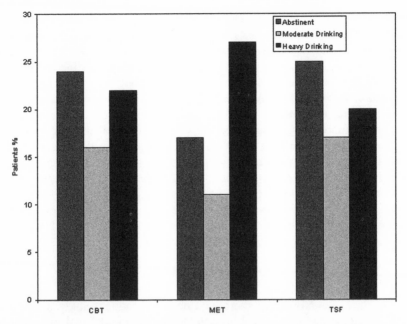

FIGURE 3.1. Project MATCH (1998b). Percentage of patients with drinking outcome at 12 weeks by treatment condition. CBT: cognitive-behavioral therapy; MET: motivational enhancement therapy; TSF: 12-step facilitation therapy. Moderate drinking is no more than 2 days when men reported consuming five drinks and women reported three drinks, or no more than 2 weeks with women reporting 11 and men reporting 14 total drinks.

tensity may explain these results since benefits dissipated soon after treatment ended, and the difference between MET, TSF, and CBT only appeared toward the end of the 12 weeks, when MET patients were no longer in treatment. The authors suggest that these results lead to a recommendation of CBT or TSF as treatments of choice if there is a need to quickly reduce heavy drinking and alcohol-related consequences.

The Project MATCH Research Group (1998a) also reported that reductions in drinking found at the 1-year outcome were maintained at 3 years. In Months 37 to 39, 30% of patients were abstinent, and those who did report drinking had been abstinent on average two thirds of the time in the past 2 years. There were few treatment differences, even though TSF did show the same slight advantage at 3-year outcome that it did at 1-year outcome on the measure of total abstinence. In regard to the matching hypotheses, clients high in anger had better outcome in MET compared to CBT or TSF at both 1- and 3-year outcome, whereas patients low in anger did better in either CBT or TSF.

In another report from Project MATCH, Longabaugh, Wirtz, Zweben, and Stout (1998)[3] found that TSF was more effective at 3-year outcome than MET for patients with networks supportive of drinking. The TSF treatment had as one of its primary aims getting the patient involved in AA, a network of people with the shared goal of supporting and sustaining abstinence. Indeed, AA involvement was a mediator of the TSF treatment effect, in that patients assigned to TSF attended AA more, and AA involvement was related to better 3-year drinking outcome.

Other important findings were a report on the actual costs of delivering the three treatments in the Project MATCH group within the research study and an estimate of the cost of delivering the treatments within regular clinic settings (Cisler, Holder, Longabaugh, Stout, & Zweben, 1998). Average cost per patient was $512 for MET, $750 for TSF, and $788 for CBT. MET was only 4 sessions in length compared with the 12 sessions of CBT or TSF, but there were no differences between the briefer and longer treatments in 1-year posttreatment outcomes (Project MATCH, 1997).

Cocaine

The results of the NIDA Collaborative Cocaine Treatment Study, a multisite randomized clinical trial of psychosocial treatments of 487 patients with cocaine dependence, were published in 1999 (Crits-Christoph et al., 1999).[4] Five research sites examined whether professional psychotherapy (plus group drug counseling) added to the benefits of group drug counseling (GDC) alone and were superior to the benefits of individual drug counseling (IDC) (plus group drug counseling). The psychotherapies were CBT and psychodynamic supportive-expressive (SE) psychotherapy. All treatments were manualized. SE was a focal psychodynamic psychotherapy that views the problems associated with the use of cocaine and with its cessation in the context of understanding the person and interpersonal relationship difficulties. Cognitive Therapy of Substance Abuse/Dependence was based on Beck's cognitive model. IDC followed a manual with specific stages, tasks, and goals based on the 12-step philosophy. GDC was designed to educate patients about the stages of recovery from addiction, to strongly encourage participation in 12-step programs, and to provide a supportive group atmosphere for initiating abstinence and alternative lifestyle. Treatment lasted for 6 months. More specific details about the study design can be found elsewhere (Crits-Christoph et al., 1997).

---

3. This paper found that TSF was more effective at 3-year outcome than MET for patients with networks supportive of drinking. Patients assigned to TSF attended AA more, and AA involvement was related to better 3-year drinking outcome.

4. This article reports the results of the NIDA Collaborative Cocaine Study, a multisite randomized clinical trial of psychosocial treatments of 487 patients with DSM-IV cocaine dependence. Individual drug counseling (IDC) plus group drug counseling (GDC) showed significantly better drug use outcome than Cognitive Therapy + GDC or SE therapy + GDC or GDC alone despite higher attrition rates for IDC.

All treatments showed significant improvements in subjects' cocaine use in last 30 days. Cocaine use improved from a mean of 10.4 days at baseline to a mean of 3.4 days at 12 months. IDC plus GDC had significantly lower days cocaine use than CT plus GDC or SE plus GDC. In addition, IDC had lower average drug use over the course of the 12-month assessment period. IDC plus GDC was significantly better than SE plus GDC and CT plus GDC, and significantly better than GDC alone. No difference was found between GDC alone and SE plus GDC and CT plus GDC (Crits-Christoph et al., 1997).

By Month 6, 39% of the available patients in the IDC plus GDC condition reported use of cocaine in the past month, whereas 57% of patients in CT plus GDC, 49% in SE plus GDC, and 52% in GDC alone reported use. The results, given in terms of percentage of patients using cocaine by treatment condition by month, can be found in Figure 3.2.

These better drug outcome results were found for patients in IDC even though they attended fewer sessions than patients in CBT and SE (IDC + GDC mean = 12, CBT + GDC = 16, SE + GDC = 16). The treatments did not differ

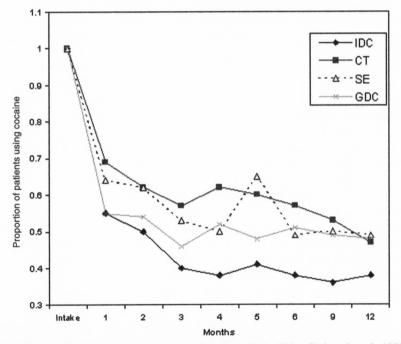

FIGURE 3.2 NIDA Collaborative Cocaine Treatment Study (Crits-Christoph et al., 1999). Adjusted proportion of patients in each treatment condition that reported any cocaine use in the past 30 days. At intake, all patients had used in the past month. Months 1–12 proportion used adjusted for site, intake number of days used, intake psychiatric severity, and intake CPI score. CT: cognitive therapy; GDC: group drug counseling; IDC: individual drug counseling; SE: supportive-expressive therapy.

on the average number of group sessions attended with patients in all treatments attending about 9 group sessions. In addition, IDC was better than SE on another important outcome, reducing overall HIV risk and, particularly, sexual risk behaviors (Crits-Christoph et al., 1999).

In trying to understand these results, a number of possible explanations were explored. There was no evidence that, for IDC plus GDC, minority therapists had better ASI Drug Use Composite outcomes with minority patients, nor that counselors in recovery from addiction had better outcomes. In addition, data on the quality of the therapeutic relationship revealed uniformly high ratings in all three individual treatments and no significant differences between them. We believe that IDC, with its clear and focused message of stopping drug use, provided patients with defined tasks and coping strategies that may be particularly helpful in initiating abstinence. In addition, there may have been a synergistic, combined effect for the GDC and IDC treatment components since they share similar goals and philosophy.

Two interaction, or treatment matching, hypotheses were also examined in the study reported in Crits-Christoph (1999). There was no evidence supporting the hypothesis that CBT, a more structured, didactic approach, was better than SE for patients with higher levels of sociopathy. It has also been hypothesized by the study investigators that the professional psychotherapies would show an advantage when patients had concurrent psychiatric problems or disorders. However, there was no evidence of a difference in the efficacy of the treatments by level of psychiatric severity.

The findings of this study were surprising for two reasons. First, it is rare to find one treatment significantly better than another treatment in psychotherapy research if the comparison treatment is credible. Second, previous literature had shown added benefits of professional psychotherapy (including cognitive therapy) compared with IDC for opiate-dependent individuals on methadone (Woody, Luborsky, et al., 1983; Woody, McLellan, Luborsky, & O'Brien, 1995). In addition, since the NIDA Collaborative Cocaine Treatment Study began, two studies of cocaine dependence have reported drug counseling to be less efficacious than either an incentive-based treatment (Higgins et al., 1993) or standard CBT (Maude-Griffin et al., 1998). Figure 3.3 compares the results of CBT and drug counseling (DC) in these two treatment studies with the results of the NIDA Collaborative Study, using a common outcome measure (percentage of intent-to-treat sample achieving at least 1 month of abstinence).

Although there are a variety of important differences between these studies, what is particularly striking is the differences in performance of the drug counseling conditions. Although Maude-Griffin et al. (1998) reported that CBT ($n = 59$) was superior to DC ($n = 69$), and the NIDA Collaborative Cocaine Treatment Study reported that DC ($n = 121$) was superior to CBT ($n = 119$), it is clear that this difference was not a function of the CBT faring poorly in the NIDA Collaborative Cocaine Treatment Study (it actually did slightly better than in Maude-Griffin et al., 1998). The DC condition in the NIDA Collabora-

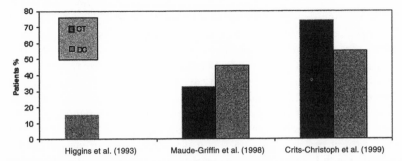

FIGURE 3.3 Percentage of randomized patients (intent-to-treat sample) who achieved at least 1 month of abstinence in three treatment studies of cocaine dependence. CT: cognitive-behavioral therapy; DC: drug counseling.

tive Cocaine Treatment Study produced results far better than were found in the other two studies. A next important step would be to understand what is particularly potent about the IDC and GDC combination offered in this study and to compare it with drug counseling as it is practiced in the community. Interestingly, the focus on the cognitive components of drug counseling, relapse prevention techniques, which are often now a part of DC in the community, were excluded from the IDC treatment in this study to allow for the comparison with CT. This potent IDC was a more straightforward 12-step behavioral approach than may be offered in usual DC.

An additional clinical trial treatment for cocaine-dependent patients continues to raise the question of whether more or intensive treatment is necessarily better. Gottheil, Weinstein, Sterling, Lundy, and Serota (1998) compared the follow-up outcome of an intensive group treatment program (3 hours of group treatment 3 times per week) with weekly individual outpatient counseling and once weekly individual plus one weekly group session for cocaine-dependent individuals. A little more than half of the 862 patients (57%) invited to participate enrolled in the study. There were no significant differences for the 447 patients on drug outcome among the three treatment conditions at 9-month follow-up, suggesting no additional benefit for the more intensive treatment.

NATURALISTIC STUDIES

The national Drug Abuse Treatment Outcome Studies (DATOS; Simpson et al., 1999),[5] a report of the effectiveness of currently available treatment pro-

---

5. The national Drug Abuse Treatment Outcome Studies (DATOS) assessed a total of 1,605 cocaine-dependent patients admitted to long-term residential programs, outpatient drug-free programs, and short-term inpatient programs. Only 23.5% of patients reported weekly cocaine use in the year following discharge from treatment, and reductions were also found in alcohol use and criminal activity. Outcome was related to treatment intensity and level of problem severity.

grams for cocaine-dependence in the community, assessed a total of 1,605 cocaine dependent patients: 542 admitted to 19 long-term residential programs, 458 admitted to 24 outpatient drug-free programs, and 605 admitted to 12 short-term inpatient programs. Only one quarter (23.5%) of patients reported weekly cocaine use in the year following discharge from treatment, and reductions were also found in alcohol use and criminal activity. Patients were rated at intake on their level of problem severity based on seven variables reflecting both severity of drug addiction (multiple drug use, alcohol dependence) and other concurrent psychologic and social problems (concurrent anxiety and depression, unemployed, low social support, no insurance, criminal involvement). Not surprisingly, patients with low levels of problem severity had the lowest relapse rates and did well in all treatment types. The worst relapse rates were found for the most severe users and those who left treatment early.

For patients with medium-level severity ratings, and especially those with high severity ratings, longer retention in treatment (>90 days in outpatient or residential treatment or >21 days in short-term inpatient) led to 50% fewer patients relapsing. However, patients with medium-level problems did equally well in the 90 days of outpatient treatment and the residential treatment. This is important since outpatient treatment had significantly lower costs. The most severe patients who stayed in the residential treatment for more than 90 days did better than most severe patients in the outpatient programs despite longer retention. Interestingly, a fourth of the sample returned to treatment in the 1-year follow-up, but this did not impact the relapse rates and did not vary by treatment type. Only 26% of the short-term inpatient patients accessed further treatment, though all patients were recommended to do so at the time of discharge (Simpson et al., 1999).

NEW APPLICATIONS OF TREATMENT APPROACHES

Two other studies have expanded work on the community reinforcement approach (CRA; Abbott, Weller, Delaney, & Moore, 1998; Smith, Meyers, & Delaney, 1998). This is a behavioral intervention focused on the environmental contingencies that can play a role in encouraging or discouraging abstinence from drugs or alcohol. It uses social, familial, recreational, and vocational reinforcers to assist reduction in substance use and often involves the patient's family members in treatment. Smith et al. (1998) found that community reinforcement showed better drinking outcomes in follow-up than standard care (shelter services, individual alcohol counseling sessions, on-site AA meetings) for homeless alcohol-dependent individuals, even though both groups showed improvements. There were no significant differences between the standard and CRA care on nondrinking outcomes. This was the first test of CRA with a homeless population.

In addition, in the first clinical trial of CRA with opiate addicts in methadone maintenance, Abbott et al. (1998) found that CRA led to more patients (89%) having 3 consecutive weeks free from opiates than patients in standard treatment (78%) and lower drug composite scores. However, there were no treatment condition differences on overall percentage of clean urine samples, number of patients 8, 12, and 16 weeks opiate-free, or any other problem areas (e.g., family, employment, level of depression). These findings suggest that CRA might help in initiation of early abstinence. Both these studies suggest that CRA approaches are promising even without the voucher system, or paying patients for clean urine samples (Higgins et al., 1993), which many clinics may have difficulty implementing.

PREDICTORS AND MEDIATORS OF OUTCOME

More and more evidence is pointing to the importance of involvement in self-help groups (AA or Narcotics Anonymous) as a mediator of improvement in substance abuse treatment. A recent study by Humphreys, Huebsch, Finney, and Moos (1999) found that the theoretical orientation of the substance abuse program influences both the proportion of patients that participate in self-help groups and the amount of benefit they derive from them. Patients treated in 12-step and eclectic programs attended more self-help than patients in cognitive-behaviorally oriented programs. In addition, as the degree of the program's emphasis on 12-step-approaches increased, the relationship between 12-step participation and drug use and psychologic outcome became stronger. The authors suggest that 12-step-oriented programs may enhance the effectiveness of 12-step self-help programs. This is very important in light of the findings of both the NIDA Collaborative Cocaine Study (Crits-Christoph et al., 1997) and Project MATCH (1998a, 1998b).

CONCLUSIONS

The good news from 1998 and 1999 is that evidence for the efficacy of several psychosocial treatments for substance abuse has been reported. Clinicians and researchers, however, continue to be surprised and disappointed by the lack of research evidence that patients can be matched to treatment based on how they present at intake. It is intuitively appealing and seems to make clinical sense. Project MATCH (1997) was specifically designed to examine patient-treatment matching and the NIDA Collaborative Cocaine Study (Crits-Christoph et al., 1997) included two matching hypotheses, but neither study found support for any of these matching hypotheses (with the exception of low-psychiatric-severity patients at 1-year follow-up).

The results of the DATOS study (Simpson et al., 1999), however, suggested that patients can be matched to type of program based on the severity of their drug use (e.g., use of multiple drugs, alcohol dependence) and other social or psychologic problems (criminal involvement, unemployment, or concurrent depression). The patients with these more severe problems benefited relatively more from intensive residential programs compared to outpatient programs, while patients with moderately severe problems fared equally well in both if they stayed in outpatient treatment at least 90 days.

It has been surprising that the psychotherapies, such as CBT or SE, that have been so helpful in treating anxiety and depression did not prove more effective than the 12-step approaches for those patients with higher psychiatric severity in either the NIDA study or Project MATCH. Perhaps the potency of the drug or alcohol and drug- or alcohol-related problems overwhelm the power of CBT and other treatments to address depression, anxiety, or other problems until the drug or alcohol use has stopped. These other treatments might be effective in later stages of recovery targeting psychiatric symptoms and other social and interpersonal problems that many substance abusers face even after they quit drugs or alcohol.

Several studies have pointed to the importance of 12-step involvement as a primary or adjunctive aspect of substance dependence treatment. The 3-year outcome for Project MATCH (1998a), the individual drug counseling advantage in the NIDA study, and the separate study by Humphreys et al. (1999) all highlight in one way or another the role of 12-step-oriented treatment. It will be important to understand the active ingredients of these 12-step-oriented approaches. What is it about them that is helpful: A new social network not based around substance or alcohol use? Sharing with others with similar problems? Specific steps about what to do when the person feels like using? All of the above? It may be helpful to work on interventions that address the concerns some patients have about self-help that prevents them from attending. Despite the potency of drugs and alcohol, psychosocial interventions have the power to change lives.

RECOMMENDED READING

Certain of the references below are of particular importance. We highlight Longabaugh et al. (1998) and, especially, Crits-Christoph et al. (1999), Project MATCH (1998a, 1998b), and Simpson et al. (1999).

REFERENCES

Abbott, P. J., Weller, S. B., Delaney, H. D., & Moore, B. A. (1998). Community reinforcement approach in the treatment of opiate addicts. *American Journal of Drug and Alcohol Abuse, 24*(1), 17–30.
Cisler, R., Holder, H. D., Longabaugh, R., Stout, R. L., & Zweben, A. (1998). Actual and

estimated replication costs for alcohol treatment modalities: Case study from project MATCH. *Journal of Studies on Alcohol, 59,* 503–512.

Crits-Christoph, P., Siqueland, L., Blaine, J., et al. (1997). The NIDA Collaborative Cocaine Treatment Study: Rationale and methods. *Archives of General Psychiatry, 54,* 721–726.

Crits-Christoph, P., Siqueland, L., Blaine, J., et al. (1999). Psychosocial treatments for cocaine dependence. *Archives of General Psychiatry, 56,* 493–502.

Gottheil, E., Weinstein, S. P., Sterling, R. C,, Lundy, A., & Serota, R. D. (1998). A randomized controlled study of the effectiveness of intensive outpatient treatment for cocaine dependence. *Psychiatric Services, 49*(6), 782–787.

Higgins, S. T., Budney, A. J., Bickel, W. K., et al. (1993). Achieving cocaine abstinence with a behavioral approach. *American Journal of Psychiatry, 150,* 763–769.

Humphreys, K., Huebsch, P. D., Finney, J. W., & Moos, R. H. (1999). A comparative evaluation of substance abuse treatment: V. Substance abuse treatment can enhance the effectiveness of self-help groups. *Alcoholism, Clinical and Experimental Research, 23*(3), 558–563.

Longabaugh, R. L., Wirtz, P. W., Zweben, A., & Stout, R. L. (1998). Network support for drinking, Alcoholics Anonymous and long-term matching effects. *Addiction, 93*(9), 1313–1333.

Maude-Griffin, P. M., Hohenstein, J. M., et al. (1998). Superior efficacy of cognitive-behavioral therapy for urban crack cocaine abusers: Main and matching effects. *Journal of Consulting and Clinical Psychology, 66,* 832–837.

National Institute on Drug Abuse Household Survey. (1996). *Substance Abuse and Mental Health Services Administration/Office of Applied Statistics.* Rockville, MD: National Institute on Drug Abuse, U.S. Department of Health and Human Services.

Project MATCH Research Group. (1997). Matching Alcoholism Treatments to Client Heterogeneity: Project MATCH post-treatment drinking outcomes. *Journal of Studies on Alcohol, 58,* 7–29.

Project MATCH Research Group. (1998a). Matching alcoholism treatments to client heterogeneity: Project MATCH three-year drinking outcomes. *Alcoholism, Clinical and Experimental Research, 22*(6), 1300–1311.

Project MATCH Research Group. (1998b). Matching alcoholism treatments to client heterogeneity: Treatment main effects and matching effects on drinking during treatment. *Journal of Studies on Alcohol, 59,* 631–639.

Regier, D. A., Farmer, M. E., Rae, D. S., et al. (1990). Comorbidity of mental disorders with alcohol and other drug abuse: Results from the epidemiologic catchment area (ECA) study. *Journal of the American Medical Association, 264,* 2511–2518.

Simpson, D. D., Joe, G. W., Fletcher, B. W., et al. (1999). A national evaluation of treatment outcomes for cocaine dependence. Psychosocial treatments for cocaine dependence. *Archives of General Psychiatry, 56,* 507–514.

Smith, J. E., Meyers, R. J., & Delaney, H. D. (1998). The community reinforcement approach with homeless alcohol-dependent individuals. *Journal of Consulting and Clinical Psychology, 66*(3), 541–548.

Woody, G. E., Luborsky, L., McLellan, A. T., et al. (1983). Psychotherapy for opiate addicts: Does it help? *Archives of General Psychiatry, 40,* 639–645.

Woody, G. E., McLellan, A. T., Luborsky, L., & O'Brien, C. P. (1995). Psychotherapy in community-based methadone programs—A validation study. *American Journal of Psychiatry, 152,* 1302–1308.

Chapter 4

Drug Therapy
for Alcohol Dependence

Robert M. Swift, M.D., Ph.D.

Alcohol dependence is a chronic disorder that results from a variety of genetic, psychosocial, and environmental factors (Morse & Flavin, 1992). As defined by the American Psychiatric Association (1994) in the *Diagnostic and Statistical Manual of Mental Disorders*, it is characterized by increased tolerance of the effects of alcohol, impaired control over drinking, and continued drinking despite adverse consequences (Table 4.1). Alcohol dependence affects nearly 10% of the population and results in social problems, considerable morbidity and mortality, and high healthcare costs (McGinnis & Foege, 1993; Rice, 1993).

Alcohol dependence is treated by medical, psychological, and social interventions that reduce or eliminate the desire to drink and the harmful effects of alcohol. Treatment usually consists of two phases: detoxification and rehabilitation. Detoxification ameliorates the symptoms and signs of withdrawal; rehabilitation helps the patient avoid future problems with alcohol. Most rehabilitative treatments are psychosocial, consisting of individual and group therapy, residential treatment in alcohol-free settings, and self-help groups such as Alcoholics Anonymous. Almost all programs advocate complete abstinence from alcohol. Although psychosocial treatments are effective in reducing alcohol consumption and in maintaining abstinence in many patients, 40% to 70% of patients resume drinking within a year after treatment (Finney, Hahn, & Moos, 1996).

There is increasing interest in drug therapy for alcohol dependence (Chick & Erickson, 1996; Institute of Medicine, 1990; Litten, Allen, & Fertig, 1996). The rationale for such therapy is based on several premises. First, advances in

TABLE 4.1. Criteria for Alcohol Dependence[a]

The diagnosis of alcohol dependence requires at least three of the following conditions during a 12-month period:

- Tolerance, that is, the need for increased amounts of alcohol in order to achieve intoxication or another desired effect, or a markedly diminished effect with use of the same amount of alcohol.
- Characteristic withdrawal symptoms, or the ingestion of alcohol to relieve or avoid withdrawal
- Ingestion of alcohol in larger amounts or over a longer period than intended
- Persistent desire or one or more unsuccessful attempts to reduce or to control alcohol ingestion
- Expenditure of much time in activities necessary to get and drink alcohol, or to recover from its effects
- Abandonment of important social, occupational, or recreational activities because of alcohol ingestion
- Continued alcohol ingestion despite the knowledge of having a persistent or recurrent social, psychological, or physical problem that is caused or exacerbated by it

[a]Adapted from the *Diagnostic and Statistical Manual of Mental Disorders* (APA, 1994).

neurobiology have identified neurotransmitter systems that initiate and maintain the drinking of alcohol. Pharmacologic modification of these neurotransmiters or their receptors may modify dependence. Second, new drugs that reduce alcohol consumption in animals may also reduce consumption in humans. Third, the development of drugs for the treatment of addictive disorders, such as nicotine and opioid dependence, suggests that it may be possible to develop drugs for the treatment of alcohol dependence.

In the United States, the Food and Drug Administration (FDA) has approved two drugs, disulfiram (Antabuse, Wyeth–Ayerst, Philadelphia) and naltrexone (ReVia, Dupont Merck, Wilmington, DE), for the treatment of alcohol dependence. Acamprosate (Campral, Lipha, Lyons, France, and Merck, Darmstadt, Germany), approved in several European countries, is being tested in the United States. Tiapride (marketed by various manufacturers) is also approved in several European countries. Other drugs marketed as mood stabilizers, sedatives, anxiolytics, and antidepressants have been used to treat alcohol dependence. This review discusses the putative mechanisms of action of these drugs and their efficacy.

THE NEUROBEHAVIORAL ASPECTS OF ALCOHOL DEPENDENCE

Alcohol is a drug with complex behavioral effects that can be pleasurable or unpleasant, stimulating or sedating. The predominant effects depend on the dose, the length of time after ingestion, whether ingestion is chronic or inter-mittent, the drinker's expectations, the setting in which alcohol is consumed, the drinker's personality, and his or her genetic predisposition to alcohol de-pendence. Alcohol affects several brain neurotransmitters, including dopamine, γ-aminobutyric acid, glutamate, serotonin, adenosine, norepinephrine, and opioid peptides, and their receptors (Chick & Erickson, 1996; Litten et al., 1996). Several neurobehavioral effects of alcohol have been related to the de-velopment of alcohol dependence (Table 4.2). These effects and their associ-ated neurotransmitters are potential targets for drug therapy to treat dependence.

The pleasurable and stimulant effects of alcohol are mediated by a dopa-minergic pathway projecting from the ventral tegmental area to the nucleus accumbens (Koob & Weiss, 1992; Samson & Hodge, 1993). Repeated exces-sive alcohol ingestion sensitizes this pathway and leads to the development of dependence (Wise & Bozarth, 1987; Robinson & Berridge, 1993). Drugs that target this dopamine system may reduce the reinforcing effects of alcohol and thereby reduce alcohol consumption. Similarly, drugs that increase the aver-sive effects of alcohol may reduce consumption. People who are more sensi-tive to the sedative and aversive effects of alcohol appear less likely to drink heavily and to develop alcohol dependence (Schuckit, 1994). Drugs that re-duce the acute and chronic symptoms of alcohol withdrawal may treat depen-dence by reducing the need for alcohol-dependent patients to ingest alcohol to avoid this state (Littleton & Little, 1994). Long-term exposure to alcohol causes adaptive changes in several neurotransmitter systems, including down-regula-tion of inhibitory neuronal γ-aminobutyric acid receptors (Suzdak, Schwartz, Skolnick, & Paul, 1986), up-regulation of excitatory glutamate receptors (Hoffman et al., 1990), and increased central norepinephrine activity (Linnoila, 1987). Discontinuation of alcohol ingestion leaves this excitatory state unop-posed, resulting in the nervous system hyperactivity and dysfunction that char-acterize alcohol withdrawal.

TABLE 4.2. Neurobehavioral Effects of Alcohol Associated
with Alcohol Dependence

Behavioral Property of Alcohol	Effect on Promoting or Inhibiting Alcohol Use
Stimulation, induction of pleasure, positive reinforcement	Promotes initial ingestion, maintains alcohol use
Sedation	May promote or inhibit alcohol ingestion
Aversion	Protects against alcohol ingestion
Tolerance	Promotes ingestion; larger amounts required for effect
Withdrawal	Promotes ingestion to diminish unpleasant symptoms
Craving	Promotes ingestion
Self-medication (anxiolytic, tension-reducing effect)	Promotes ingestion to alleviate psychological distress

People who drink alcohol over long periods and excessively also have craving, defined as the conscious desire or urge to drink alcohol. Intense craving leads to a preoccupation with alcohol and increases the probability of drinking (Anton, Moak, & Latham, 1995). Craving can occur in several circumstances: before alcohol ingestion, during alcohol ingestion, during acute withdrawal, and during exposure to the sight or smell of alcohol long after drinking has stopped. Craving has been linked to dopaminergic, serotonergic, and opioid systems that mediate positive reinforcement and to γ-aminobutyric acid, glutamatergic, and noradrenergic systems that mediate withdrawal (Littleton & Little, 1994). Reductions in craving are associated with longer abstinence (Anton, Moak, & Latham, 1996; Rohsenow et al., 1992).

Finally, it is proposed that some persons with psychiatric disorders become dependent on alcohol as a result of self-medication with alcohol to reduce psychiatric symptoms and distress (Khantzian, 1985). Alcohol dependence is common among patients with schizophrenia, panic disorder, and depression (Regier et al., 1990). Drugs that effectively treat the underlying psychiatric disorder may reduce the impetus for alcohol ingestion.

DRUG TREATMENT FOR ALCOHOL DEPENDENCE

Most studies of drug treatment for alcoholism compare differences in drinking outcomes between treatment with the drug and with placebo in recently abstinent patients who are also receiving psychosocial therapy. Typical outcomes include increases in abstinence, expressed as the proportion of patients remaining abstinent or the length of time to the loss of abstinence (relapse), and reductions in the quantity or frequency of drinking, expressed as the number of drinking days or the number of drinks per drinking day. Although abstinence is the more stringent outcome and is preferred, reductions in consumption can nevertheless reduce alcohol-related morbidity. The drugs discussed below have been evaluated in double-blind, placebo-controlled clinical trials (Table 4.3).

Aversive Drugs

Alcohol metabolism is a two-stage process. Ethanol is converted to acetaldehyde by alcohol dehydrogenase, and acetaldehyde is then converted to acetate by aldehyde dehydrogenase (Figure 4.1). For most people ingesting alcohol, acetaldehyde is metabolized rapidly and efficiently, so that it does not accumulate. When it does accumulate, it causes tachycardia, flushing, diaphoresis, dyspnea, nausea, and vomiting. Inhibition of aldehyde dehydrogenase by disulfiram, an irreversible inhibitor, or calcium carbimide, a shorter acting, reversible inhibitor, causes the accumulation of sufficient acetaldehyde to cause

TABLE 4.3. Drugs with Some Evidence of Efficacy in Patients
with Alcohol Dependence[a]

Drug Approved[b]	Class	Proposed Mechanism of Action in Alcohol Dependence	Neurotransmitter System Affected
Acamprosate	NMDA and GABA$_A$ receptor modulator	Reduces unpleasant effects of alcohol abstinence, reduces craving	Glutamate, GABA
Calcium carbimide	Aversive agent	Increases aversive effects of alcohol by increasing acetaldehyde	Unknown
Disulfiram	Aversive agent	Increases aversive effects of alcohol by increasing acetaldehyde	Dopamine (?)
Naltrexone	Opioid antagonist	Reduces pleasurable, stimulating effects of alcohol, reduces craving	Opioid
Tiapride	Dopamine antagonist	Reduces pleasurable, stimulating effects of alcohol, reduces anxiety	Dopamine
Experimental Bromocriptine	Dopamine agonist	Reduces unpleasant effects of abstinence	Dopamine
Buspirone	Anxiolytic	Reduces anxiety in anxious alcohol-dependent patients	Serotonin
Carbamazepine	Mood stabilizer, anticonvulsant	Reduces unpleasant effects of alcohol withdrawal and abstinence	Unknown
γ-Hydroxybutyric acid	Sedative	Reduces unpleasant effects of alcohol withdrawal and abstinence	GABA
Nalmetene	Opioid antagonist	Reduces pleasurable, stimulating effects of alcohol, reduces craving	Opioid
SSRIs	Anti-depressant	Reduce depression and anxiety associated with alcohol dependence in depressed patients	Serotonin
Tricyclic antidepressants	Anti-depressant	Reduce depression and anxiety associated with alcohol dependence in depressed patients	Serotonin, norepinephrine

[a]NMDA denotes N-methyl-D-asparate, GABA denotes γ-aminobutyric acid, and SSRIs denotes selective serotonin-reuptake inhibitors.
[b]These drugs have been approved by regulatory agencies in the United States, Canada, or Europe for the treatment of alcohol dependence.

symptoms. The possibility of having these unpleasant symptoms provides a deterrent to alcohol ingestion.

Although disulfiram has been reported to be an effective treatment for alcohol dependence in case reports and open-label studies, placebo-controlled clinical trials have been inconclusive (Hughes & Cook, 1997; Peachey & Annis,

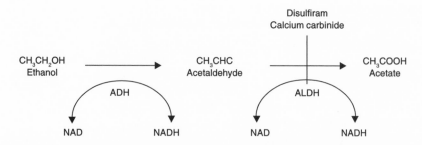

FIGURE 4.1. The site of action of disulfiram and calcium carbimide in the metabolism of ethanol. ADH: alcohol dehydrogenase, ALDH: aldehyde dehydrogenase, NAD: nicotinamide adenine dinucleotide, and NADH: reduced NAD.

1989). In the most rigorous and best-controlled double-blind treatment study, in which 605 alcohol-dependent men were treated with 250 mg of disulfiram daily, 1 mg of disulfiram daily (a pharmacologically ineffective dose), or no drug for a year, there were no differences in rates of abstinence or the length of time to a first drink among the three groups (Fuller et al., 1986). Only men receiving 250 mg of disulfiram who ingested alcohol and became ill subsequently drank less alcohol than those in the other two groups. The authors concluded that disulfiram neither improves the rate of continuous abstinence nor delays the resumption of drinking, but that it may reduce drinking after relapse.

In spite of its lack of efficacy as compared with placebo, some physicians and patients believe that disulfiram is an effective psychological deterrent to drinking. The usual dose of disulfiram is 250 mg per day, although doses of 125 mg to 1000 mg are sometimes given, depending on side effects and response. Some patients take disulfiram only when they are at high risk for relapse; others take it continuously. Administration of disulfiram under direct observation reportedly increases its effectiveness (Chick et al., 1992).

Patients taking disulfiram must be aware of the danger of consuming alcohol in beverages, foods, over-the-counter medications, or mouthwashes. Disulfiram inhibits the metabolism of several medications, notably anticoagulant drugs, phenytoin, and isoniazid, thereby exaggerating their actions and toxic effects. It should be given cautiously to patients with liver disease and is contraindicated in pregnant women and patients with ischemic heart disease. Disulfiram can cause hepatitis, and liver-function tests should therefore be performed regularly during treatment.

Calcium carbimide (Temposil, Lederle, Markham, ON, Canada), previously available in Canada and Australia, was withdrawn from the market by its manufacturer. It has not been studied as extensively as disulfiram. Like disulfiram, it also has been no more effective than placebo in clinical trials. In a 4-month, randomized, double-blind, crossover study of calcium carbimide and placebo in 128 alcohol-dependent patients, those who completed the study had lower alcohol consumption and increased rates of abstinence during both the placebo and calcium carbimide treatment periods (Peachey et al., 1989). The authors concluded that calcium carbimide acted as a psychological deterrent to drinking, because even while patients were receiving placebo, the possibility that they might be taking the active drug reduced alcohol ingestion. However, the lack of a group that received no medication makes these conclusions speculative. Calcium carbimide has few side effects, but it has been associated with leukocytosis and hypothyroidism.

Opioid Antagonists

The observation that μ-opioid (morphine-like) agonists increased alcohol consumption and that μ-opioid antagonists reduced alcohol consumption in animals (Froelich, Harts, Lumeng, & Li, 1990; Hubbell et al., 1986) led to clinical trials of naltrexone in patients with alcohol dependence. It has been proposed that naltrexone reduces drinking and increases abstinence by reducing the positively reinforcing, pleasurable effects of alcohol and by reducing the craving for alcohol. Naltrexone and other μ-opioid antagonists block the alcohol-induced release of dopamine in the nucleus accumbens (Benjamin, Grant, & Pohorecky, 1993; Gessa, Muntoni, Collu, Vargiu, & Mereu, 1985). Social drinkers report less positive and more sedative and unpleasant effects of alcohol when taking naltrexone (Swift, Whelihan, Kuznetsov, Buongiorno, & Hsuing, 1994). Patients with alcoholism who drink during treatment with naltrexone report experiencing less alcohol "high" and are less likely to progress to heavy drinking (Volpicelli, Watson, King, Sherman, & O'Brien, 1995). Naltrexone also reduces the craving for alcohol in both alcoholic patients (Monti et al., in press) and social drinkers (Davidson, Swift, & Fitz, 1996).

Several double-blind, placebo-controlled trials have found that naltrexone is efficacious when combined with psychosocial treatments for alcohol dependence. In a 12-week, placebo-controlled, randomized clinical trial of 50 mg of naltrexone daily in 70 alcohol-dependent men receiving outpatient psychotherapy, the patients receiving naltrexone had significantly fewer drinking days than those given placebo (4% vs. 14% of study days), and fewer later resumed heavy drinking, defined as consuming five or more drinks in a day (23% vs. 54% of the men; Volpicelli, Alterman, Hayashida, & O'Brien, 1992). In a double-blind study of 97 alcohol-dependent men and women given 50 mg of naltrexone or placebo per day and assigned either to therapy targeted to increasing individual coping skills and relapse prevention or to supportive therapy for 12 weeks, alcohol consumption was lower and the abstinence rate was higher among the naltrexone-treated patients (O'Malley et al., 1992). Fewer than half the patients in the naltrexone group resumed heavy drinking, as compared with more than 80% of those in the placebo group. Naltrexone was most effective for patients who reported strong cravings at study entry (Jaffe et al.,

1996). An interaction between medication and psychotherapy was found, in that naltrexone increased abstinence among patients assigned to receive supportive psychotherapy but not among those assigned to psychotherapy designed primarily to increase coping skills. However, for patients taking naltrexone who drank, those who received coping-skills training were less likely to drink heavily than those who received supportive therapy.

Other studies of naltrexone found no evidence of efficacy. In a randomized trial, 108 patients with alcohol dependence and cocaine and opiate abuse received both psychosocial therapy and either placebo or 50 or 100 mg of naltrexone daily; naltrexone did not alter drinking (McCaul, Wand, Sullivan, Mumford, & Quigley, in press). Similarly, in a randomized, double-blind trial in the United Kingdom, there were no differences in drinking-related outcomes among 175 patients with alcoholism who were assigned to minimal psychosocial treatment and received either 50 mg of naltrexone per day or placebo for 12 weeks (Chick, 1996). In a randomized, double-blind, placebo-controlled trial of 50 mg of naltrexone per day or placebo in 64 patients with combined alcohol and cocaine dependence, naltrexone was no more beneficial than placebo (Hersh, Van Kirk, & Kranzler, 1998).

There are several possible reasons for the positive effects of naltrexone on drinking outcomes found in some studies and the lack of effect in others. One of the negative studies of naltrexone (Hersh et al., 1998) was probably too small to detect differences between the drug and placebo groups for a drug with a moderate effect. In two of the negative studies (McCaul et al., in press; Hersh et al., 1998), the patients abused multiple substances, which may have limited the efficacy of naltrexone. Another important variable is compliance with medication. In the negative study in the United Kingdom, naltrexone significantly decreased the total number of drinks consumed and the number of drinks per day, as compared with placebo, but only among patients who took at least 80% of the prescribed medication (Chick, 1996). The importance of compliance is supported by a U.S. study comparing naltrexone with placebo in 97 patients with alcoholism who also received weekly counseling. Those who were more compliant with naltrexone therapy were significantly less likely to report episodes of heavy drinking than those assigned to placebo (14% vs. 52%) and had fewer drinking days (2.8% vs. 11%), whereas the results among the noncompliant patients did not differ from those in the placebo group (Volpicelli et al., 1997).

For the first 90 days of abstinence, when the risk of relapse is greatest, the recommended dose of naltrexone is 50 mg once daily, but doses of 25 to 100 mg daily are sometimes used. The most common side effects are nausea (10%), headache (7%), anxiety (2%), and sedation (2%; Croop, Faulkner, & Labriola, 1997). The ingestion of naltrexone results in insensitivity to opioid drugs for 72 hours; if an opiate analgesic drug is required in an emergency, administration of a higher dose of opiates can overcome this insensitivity, but respiratory monitoring is mandatory. Although doses of 300 mg of naltrexone daily have been associated with hepatotoxic effects, such effects are rare at daily doses of 50 mg (Berg, Pettinati, & Volpicelli, 1997). Indeed, serum aminotransferase concentrations are often lower in patients given naltrexone than those given placebo, presumably because of their decreased alcohol ingestion (Jaffe et al., 1996). Nevertheless, patients with liver disease should be given naltrexone cautiously, and their liver function should be monitored periodically throughout treatment (Center for Substance Abuse Treatment, 1998).

Nalmefene, a μ- and κ-opioid antagonist, which is approved by the FDA for the reversal of opioid intoxication and overdose, is chemically similar to naltrexone but less hepatoxic (Salvato & Mason, 1994). In a 12-week clinical study of 21 patients with alcohol dependence who were given daily doses of 10 mg of nalmefene, 40 mg of nalmefene, or placebo, the higher dose nalmefene group was more abstinent than the other two groups (Mason et al., 1994).

Acamprosate

Acamprosate is thought to have agonist activity at γ-aminobutyric acid receptors (Daoust et al., 1992) and inhibitory activity at N-methyl-D-aspartate receptors (Nie, Madamba, & Siggins, 1994; Zeise, Kasparov, Capogna, & Zieglgansberger, 1993). Acamprosate normalizes the glutamatergic excitation that occurs in alcohol withdrawal and early abstinence (Samson & Harris, 1992; Tsai, Gastfriend, & Coyle, 1995). This effect may reduce craving and distress and may thus decrease the need to consume alcohol (Litten, 1996).

The observation that acamprosate reduced alcohol consumption in animals (Nalpas, Dabadic, Parot, & Paccalir, 1990; Spanagel, Holter, Allingham, Landgraf, & Zieglgansberger, 1996) led to studies in humans with alcoholism. In all but one of several European multicenter clinical trials, approximately twice as many patients given acamprosate as patients given placebo remained abstinent from alcohol during treatment periods of three months to one year (Geerings, Ansoms, & van der Brink, 1997; Ladewig, Knecht, Leher, & Fendl, 1993; Lhuintre et al., 1990; Poldrugo, 1997; Sass, Soyka, Mann, & Zieglgansberger, 1996; Soyka & Sass, 1994; Whitworth et al., 1996).

Three studies are representative of the several studies of acamprosate. In a clinical study of 85 recently abstinent patients with alcoholism who were receiving psychosocial therapy and were treated with 2,000 mg of acamprosate daily or placebo for 12 weeks, 60% of the patients receiving acamprosate remained abstinent, as compared with 22% of those receiving placebo (Lhuintre et al., 1990). In a 48-week study of 272 alcohol-dependent patients, 43% of the acamprosate group remained abstinent, as compared with 21% of the placebo group (Sass et al., 1996). The one negative study of acamprosate was a 24-week multicenter study of mildly alcohol-dependent patients in the United Kingdom, in which 20% of both the acamprosate and placebo groups remained abstinent (Chick, 1995); the lack of effectiveness of acamprosate could have been due to the mildness of the patients' alcohol dependence, however.

Acamprosate is not metabolized but is eliminated by renal excretion. It should therefore be given cautiously to patients with renal impairment. Its main side effects are diarrhea (10%) and headache (20%). The usual dose of acamprosate is 2 to 3 g per day in divided doses. Acamprosate is not yet available in the United States.

Dopaminergic Drugs

Given the theoretical importance of dopamine in the neurobiology of alcohol dependence, there is interest in dopaminergic drugs as treatments for alcohol dependence. In animals, dopamine agonists and antagonists both decrease the stimulant and positively reinforcing properties of alcohol and decrease alcohol consumption. Dopamine antagonists can block the reinforcing effects of alcohol (Broadbent, Grahame, & Cunningham, 1995); agonists may alleviate a dopamine-deficiency state (George et al., 1995). Tiapride, a dopamine D2-antagonist drug marketed in Europe as an atypical neuroleptic and anxiolytic drug, reduces the symptoms of alcohol withdrawal and is approved for the treatment of acute and chronic alcoholism (Peters & Faulds, 1994). Its efficacy in patients with alcohol dependence has been evaluated in three clinical trials. In the largest, 100 recently abstinent alcohol-dependent patients were randomly assigned to receive 300 mg of tiapride per day or placebo for 3 months. Although only 54% of subjects complied with medication for at least 1 month, those who did and who received tiapride were more likely to remain abstinent and had lower rates of use of healthcare services (Shaw et al., 1994).

The dopamine agonist bromocriptine, used in the treatment of Parkinson's disease, was initially reported to reduce drinking in patients with alcoholism (Lawford et al., 1995). However, a long-acting injectable bromocriptine preparation was no more effective than placebo in preventing relapses of drinking in 366 alcohol-dependent patients (Naranjo, Dongier, & Bremner, 1997).

Other Drugs

Several other drugs have been tested in patients with alcohol dependence, usually after they have been observed to reduce alcohol consumption in animals. Although some have reduced alcohol consumption in humans, none have been approved for the treatment of alcohol dependence.

Mood Stabilizers

Lithium reduces alcohol consumption in animals and blocks alcohol intoxication in social drinkers (Judd et al., 1977). In a double-blind, placebo-controlled study of 457 patients with alcoholism, lithium carbonate did not reduce drinking (Dorus et al., 1989). A review concluded that lithium was ineffective in treating alcohol dependence (Lejoveux & Ades, 1993).

The mood stabilizer and anticonvulsant drug carbamazepine has been used to treat alcohol withdrawal and has been reported to improve the treatment of alcohol dependence (Malcolm, Ballenger, Sturgis, & Anton, 1989). A randomized, double-blind study of 29 alcohol-dependent patients who received carbamazepine or placebo for 12 months beginning at detoxification found less drinking in those receiving carbamazepine (Mueller et al., 1997). However, the small number of patients makes the findings inconclusive.

Sedative Drugs

Although benzodiazepines and other drugs are often given to treat alcohol withdrawal, they are not given to treat alcohol dependence. Alcohol-dependent patients who receive maintenance doses of a sedative can become dependent on the sedative (Ciraulo, Sands, & Shader, 1988). The γ-aminobutyric acid agonist γ-hydroxybutyric acid reduced alcohol consumption in a double-blind clinical trial conducted in Italy (Gallimberti, Ferri, Ferrara, Fadda, & Gessa, 1992). In this 3-month outpatient study, 82 patients were randomly assigned to receive 50 mg of γ-hydroxybutyric acid per kilogram daily or placebo. Drinking was assessed on the basis of the patients' own reports and measurements of serum aminotransferase concentrations. At the end of treatment, 30.6% of the patients treated with γ-hydroxybutyric acid remained abstinent, as compared with 5.7% of the patients given placebo. Since γ-hydroxybutyric acid can be abused as a sedative, its use in maintenance therapy would be harmful in alcohol-dependent patients.

Serotonergic Drugs

Serotonin may modulate the behavioral effects of alcohol, although its effects are complex because of the presence of multiple subtypes of serotonin receptors (Kranzler & Anton, 1994; Le Marquand, Pihl, & Benkelfat, 1994; Linnoila, Eckardt, Durcan, Lister, & Martin, 1987; Sellers, Higgins, & Sobell, 1992). Selective serotonin-reuptake inhibitors, such as fluoxetine, sertaline, and citalopram, which are used clinically as antidepressant and anxiolytic drugs, increase serotonergic function and reduce alcohol consumption in animals. In trials in patients without depression who were heavy drinkers, selective serotonin-reuptake inhibitors reduced alcohol consumption by 15% to 20% (Naranjo, Poulos, Bremner, & Lanctot, 1994; Naranjo et al., 1987). Patients who are taking one of these drugs report a decreased desire and liking for alcohol (Naranjo & Bremner, 1994). However, the results in patients with diagnosed alcohol dependence have been less impressive. In a 3-week prospective study of fluoxetine, alcohol intake decreased only during the first week (Gorelick, 1993), and in a double-blind study comparing fluoxetine treatment with placebo in 101 patients, in which both groups received cognitive–behavioral psychotherapy, there was no difference in drinking between the groups (Kranzler et al., 1995).

Several serotonin-receptor agonists and antagonists that reduced alcohol consumption in animals were tested in alcohol-dependent patients. Buspirone (an anxiolytic drug that is a partial serotonin agonist at 1A and 2 receptors), ondansetron (an antagonist at serotonin-3 receptors), and ritanserin (an antagonist at serotonin-2 receptors) all reduced alcohol consumption in alcohol-drinking rats (Bruno, 1989; Collins & Myers, 1987; Knapp & Pohorecky, 1992). However, placebo-controlled clinical trials of these drugs in patients with alcohol dependence have not demonstrated efficacy for any of them (Johnson et al., 1996; Malec, Malec, Gagne, & Dongier, 1996; Sellers et al., 1994).

PATIENTS WITH PSYCHIATRIC DISORDERS

Alcohol dependence is associated with major depression, anxiety disorders, and schizophrenia (Helzer & Pryzbeck, 1988; Kessler et al., 1997; Regier et al., 1990). The relation of alcohol consumption to these illnesses is complex; it may precede the psychiatric illness or be precipitated by it. By reducing symptoms of the psychiatric illness, drug therapy may reduce the impetus for patients to medicate themselves with alcohol (Khantzian, 1985).

In patients with both alcohol dependence and major depression, antidepressant drugs combined with psychosocial treatments improve depression and, to a lesser extent, alcohol dependence. In a double-blind, placebo-controlled trial of the tricyclic antidepressant drug desipramine in 71 recently abstinent patients with alcoholism, with or without secondary depression, desipramine improved depression (Mason, Koesis, Ritvo, & Cutler, 1996). Although there were no significant differences in the rate of abstinence between the treatment groups, the depressed patients who were treated with desipramine had fewer heavy-drinking days (8% vs. 40% in the placebo group). In a double-blind, placebo-controlled trial of imipramine and weekly psychotherapy designed to prevent relapses in 69 patients with alcoholism and primary major depression or dysthymia, imipramine improved mood slightly but did not decrease drinking (McGrath et al., 1996). In a 12-week randomized, double-blind, placebo-controlled study of fluoxetine in 51 patients with major depression and alcohol dependence, fluoxetine improved depression and reduced the total number of drinks consumed during the trial by 50%, as compared with placebo (Cornelius et al., 1997).

Two studies examined the anxiolytic drug buspirone in the treatment of patients with anxiety and alcoholism, with different outcomes. In a 12-week study of 60 mg of buspirone or placebo daily in 61 patients with anxiety and alcoholism who were receiving behavioral therapy, those given buspirone remained in treatment longer and drank less than those receiving placebo (mean, 4 vs. 10 drinking days; Kranzler et al., 1994). However, in a double-blind study of 67 patients with anxiety and alcoholism, buspirone was not more effective than placebo (Malcolm et al., 1992).

RECOMMENDATIONS

Drug therapy should be considered for all patients in whom alcohol dependence is diagnosed who do not have medical contraindications to the use of the drug and who are willing to take it. Of the several drugs studied for the treatment of alcohol dependence, the evidence of efficacy is strongest for naltrexone and acamprosate. Naltrexone is currently available in the United States; acamprosate and tiapride are currently available in Europe but not in the United States.

Although disulfiram is approved for treatment of alcohol dependence in the United States and calcium carbimide was approved in Canada, there is little evidence to support the use of these aversive drugs. Still, some patients and clinicians believe that aversive drugs provide an effective psychological deterrent to drinking.

Alcohol-dependent patients with psychiatric disorders, such as depression and anxiety disorders, should be treated with drugs that are effective for the psychiatric condition. The selection of a specific drug should depend on the patient's clinical state and the pharmacokinetics of the drug. For suicidal patients, selective serotonin-reuptake inhibitors are preferred over tricyclic antidepressant drugs because of their relative lack of toxicity. Because chronic, heavy alcohol use can induce higher concentrations of hepatic metabolic enzymes, higher-than-usual doses of antidepressant drugs may be required to achieve therapeutic plasma concentrations (Mason, 1996).

Although therapy with two or more drugs with different mechanisms of action, given together or in sequence, may yield additive or synergistic benefits in patients with alcohol dependence, there is no evidence that multiple-drug therapy improves the effectiveness of treatment. Drug therapy for alcohol-dependent patients should be combined with psychosocial therapy to provide emotional support, to address the psychological and social problems associated with alcohol dependence, and to increase compliance with drug therapy. Finally, clinicians and patients should recognize that alcohol dependence is tenacious. Current drug therapies do not eliminate alcohol dependence but, rather, help to reduce drinking and achieve longer periods of abstinence for some patients.

CONCLUSIONS

In patients with alcohol dependence, drug therapy can improve the outcomes of treatment and thereby reduce morbidity and mortality and improve the quality of life. Questions remain about the optimal drug dosage, the duration of treatment, concomitant psychosocial therapy, the cost effectiveness of drug therapy, and the types of patients who will benefit most from a specific drug.

REFERENCES

American Psychiatric Association. (1994). *Diagnostic and statistical manual of mental disorders* (4th ed.). Washington, DC: Author.

Anton, R. F., Moak, D. H., & Latham, P. K. (1995). The Obsessive Compulsive Drinking Scale: A self-rated instrument for the quantification of thoughts about alcohol and drinking behavior. *Alcoholism, Clinical and Experimental Research, 19,* 92–99.

Anton, R. F., Moak, D. H., & Latham, P. K. (1995). The Obsessive Compulsive Drinking Scale: a new method of assessing outcome in alcoholism treatment studies. *Archives of General Psychiatry, 53,* 225–231. [Erratum. (1995). *Archives of General Psychiatry, 53,* 576.]

Benjamin, D., Grant, E., & Pohorecky, L. A. (1993). Naltrexone reverse ethanol-induced dopamine release in the nucleus accumbens in awake, freely moving rats. *Brain Research, 621,* 137–140.

Berg, B. J., Pettinati, H. M., & Volpicelli, J. R. (1997). A risk-benefit assessment of naltrexone in the treatment of alcohol dependence. *Drug Safety, 15,* 274–282.

Broadbent, J. G., Grahame, N. J., & Cunningham, C. L. (1995). Haloperidol prevents ethanol-stimulated locomotor activity but fails to block sensitization. *Psychopharmacology, 120,* 475–482.

Bruno, E. (1989). Buspirone in the treatment of alcoholic patients. *Psychopathology, 22*(Suppl. 1), 49–59.

Center for Subtance Abuse Treatment. (1998). Naltrexone and alcoholism treatment. Treatment improvement protocol (TIP) series 28. Rockville, MD: Center for Substance Abuse Treatment. (DHHS publication no. (SMA) 98–3206.)

Chick, J. (1995). Acamprosate as an aid in the treatment of alcoholism. *Alcohol and Alcoholism, 30,* 785–787.

Chick, J. (1996, August). UK multicentre study of naltrexone as adjunctive therapy in the treatment of alcoholism: Efficacy results. Presented at the 10th World Psychiatry Conference, Madrid, Spain.

Chick, J., & Erickson, C. K. (1996). Conference summary: Consensus Conference on Alcohol Dependence and the Role of Pharmacotherapy in Its Treatment. *Alcoholism, Clinical and Experimental Research, 20,* 391–402.

Chick, J., Gough, K., Falkowski, W., et al. (1992). Disulfiram treatment of alcoholism. *British Journal of Psychiatry, 161,* 84–89.

Ciraulo, D. A., Sands, B. F., & Shader, R. I. (1988). Critical review of liability for benzodiazepine abuse among alcoholics. *American Journal of Psychiatry, 145,* 1501–1506.

Collins, D. M., & Myers, R. D. (1987). Buspirone attenuates volitional alcohol intake in the chronically drinking monkey. *Alcohol, 4,* 49–56.

Cornelius, J. R., Salloum, I. M., Ehler, J. G., et al. (1997). Fluoxetine in depressed alcoholics: A double-blind, placebo-controlled trial. *Archives of General Psychiatry, 54,* 700–705.

Croop, R. S., Faulkner, E. B., & Labriola, D. F. (1997). The safety profile of naltrexone in the treatment of alcoholism: Results from a multicenter usage study. *Archives of General Psychiatry, 54,* 1130–1135.

Daoust, M., Legrand, E., Gewiss, M., et al. (1992). Acamprosate modulates synaptosomal GABA transmission in chronically alcoholised rats. *Pharmacology, Biochemistry and Behavior, 41,* 669–674.

Davidson, D., Swift, R. M., & Fitz, E. (1996). Naltrexone increases the latency to drink alcohol in social drinkers. *Alcoholism, Clinical and Experimental Research, 20,* 732–739.

Dorus, W., Ostrow, D. G., Anton, R., et al. (1989). Lithium treatment: Of depressed and nondepressed alcoholics. *Journal of the American Medical Association, 262,* 1646–1652.

Finney, J. W., Hahn, A. C., & Moos, R. H. (1996). The effectiveness of inpatient and outpatient treatment for alcohol abuse: The need to focus on mediators and moderators of setting effects. *Addiction, 91,* 1773–1796, 1803–1820.

Froehlich, J. C., Harts, J., Lumeng, L., & Li, T. K. (1990). Naloxone attenuates voluntary ethanol intake in rats selectively bred for high ethanol preference. *Pharmacology, Biochemistry and Behavior, 35,* 385–390.

Fuller, R. K., Branchey, L., Brightwell, D. R., et al. (1986). Disulfiram treatment of alcoholism: A Veterans Administration cooperative study. *Journal of the American Medical Association, 256,* 1449–1455.

Gallimberti, L., Ferri, M., Ferrara, S. D., Fadda, F., & Gessa, G. L. (1992). Gamma hydroxybutyric acid in the treatment of alcohol dependence: A double blind study. *Alcoholism, Clinical and Experimental Research, 16,* 673–676.

Geerings, P. J., Ansoms, C., & van der Brink, W. (1997). Acamprosate and prevention of relapse in alcoholics: Results of a randomized, placebo-controlled, double-blind study in outpatient alcoholics in the Netherlands, Belgium and Luxembourg. *European Addiction Research, 3,* 129–137.

George, S. R., Fan, T., Ng, G. Y. K., Jung, S. Y., O'Dowd, B. F., & Naranjo, C. A. (1995). Low endogenous dopamine function in brain predisposes to high alcohol preference and consumption: Reversal by increasing synaptic dopamine. *Journal of Pharmacology and Experimental Therapeutics, 273,* 373–379.

Gessa, G. L., Muntoni, F., Collu, M., Vargiu, L., & Mereu, G. (1985). Low doses of ethanol activate dopaminergic neurons in the ventral tegmental area. *Brain Research, 348,* 201–203.

Gorelick, D. A. (1993). Recent developments in alcoholism: Pharmacological treatment. *Recent Developments in Alcoholism, 11,* 413–427.

Helzer, J. E., & Pryzbeck, T. R.(1988). The co-occurrence of alcoholism with other psychiatric disorders in the general population and its impact on treatment. *Journal of Studies on Alcohol, 49,* 219–224.

Hersh, D., Van Kirk, J. R., & Kranzler, H. R. (1998). Naltrexone treatment of comorbid alcohol and cocaine use disorders. *Psychopharmacology (Berl), 139,* 44–52.

Hoffman, P. L., Rabe, C. S., Grant, K. A., Valverius, P., Hudspith, M., & Tabakoff, B. (1990). Ethanol and the NMDA receptor. *Alcohol, 7,* 229–231.

Hubbell, C. L., Czirr, S. A., Hunter, G. A., Beaman, C. M., LeCann, N. C., & Reid, L. D. (1986). Consumption of ethanol solution is potentiated by morphine and attenuated by naloxone persistently across repeated daily administrations. *Alcohol, 3,* 39–54.

Hughes, J. C., & Cook, C. C. H. (1997). The efficacy of disulfiram: A review of outcome studies. *Addiction, 92,* 381–395.

Institute of Medicine. (1990). *Broadening the base of treatment for alcohol problems: Report of a study by a committee of the Institute of Medicine. Division of Mental Health and Behavioral Medicine.* Washington, DC: National Academy Press.

Jaffe, A. J., Rounsaville, B., Chang, G., Schottenfeld, R. S., Meyer, R. E., & O'Malley, S.

S. (1996). Naltrexone, relapse prevention, and supportive therapy with alcoholics: An analysis of patient treatment matching. *Journal of Consulting Clinical Psychology, 64,* 1044–1053.

Johnson, B. A., Jasinski, D. R., Galloway, G. P., et al. (1996). Ritanserin in the treatment of alcohol dependence—a multi-center clinical trial: Ritanserin Study Group. *Psychopharmacology (Berl), 128,* 206–215.

Judd, L..L. Hubbard, B. R., Huey, L. Y., Attewell, P. A., Janowsky, D. S., & Takahashi, K. I. (1977). Lithium carbonate and ethanol induced "highs" in normal subjects. *Archives of General Psychiatry, 34,* 463–467.

Kessler, R. C., Crum, R. M., Warner, L. A., Nelson, C. B., Schulenberg, J., & Anthony, J. C. (1997). Lifetime co-occurrence of DSM-III-R alcohol abuse and dependence with other psychiatric disorders in the National Comorbidity Survey. *Archives of General Psychiatry, 54,* 313–321.

Khantzian, E. J. (1985). The self-medication hypothesis of addictive disorders: Focus on heroin and cocaine dependence. *American Journal of Psychiatry, 142,* 1259–1264.

Knapp, D. J., & Pohorecky, L. A. (1992). Zacopride, a 5HT3 receptor antagonist, reduces voluntary ethanol consumption in rats. *Pharmacology, Biochemistry, and Behavior, 41,* 847–850.

Koob, G. F., & Weiss, F. (1992). Neuropharmacology of cocaine and ethanol dependence. *Recent Developments in Alcoholism, 10,* 201–233.

Kranzler, H. R, & Anton, R. F. (1994). Implications of recent neuropsychopharmacologic research for understanding the etiology and development of alcoholism. *Journal of Consulting and Clinical Psychology, 62,* 1116–1126.

Kranzler, H. R., Burleson, J. A., Del Boca, F. K., et al. (1994). Buspirone treatment of anxious alcoholics: A placebo-controlled trial. *Archives of General Psychiatry, 51,* 720–731.

Kranzler, H. R., Burleson, J. A., Korner, P., et al. (1995). Placebo-controlled trial of fluoxetine as an adjunct to relapse prevention in alcoholics. *American Journal of Psychiatry, 152,* 391–397.

Ladewig, D., Knecht, T., Leher, P., & Fendl, A. (1993). Acamprosatcin—Stabilisierungs faktor in der Langzeitentwohnung von Alkoholabhangigen. *Therapeutische Umschau, 50,* 182–188.

Lawford, B. R., Young, R. M., Rowell, J. A., et al. (1995). Bromocriptine in the treatment of alcoholics with the D_2 dopamine receptor Al allele. *Nature Medicine, 1,* 337–341.

Lejoveux, M., & Ades, J. (1993). Evaluation of lithium treatment in alcoholism. *Alcohol and Alcoholism, 28,* 273–279.

LeMarquand, D., Pihl, R. O., & Benkelfat, C. (1994). Serotonin and alcohol intake, abuse, and dependence: Findings of animal studies. *Biological Psychiatry, 36,* 395–421.

Lhuintre, J. P., Moore, N., Tran, G., et al. (1990). Acamprosate appears to decrease alcohol intake in weaned alcoholics. *Alcohol and Alcoholism, 25,* 613–622.

Linnoila, M. (1987). NIH conference; alcohol withdrawal and noradrenergic function. *Annals of Internal Medicine, 107,* 875–889.

Linnoila, M., Eckardt, M., Durcan, M., Lister, R., & Martin, P. (1987). Interactions of serotonin with ethanol: Clinical and animal studies. *Psychopharmacology Bulletin, 23,* 452–457.

Litten, R. Z., Allen, J., & Fertig, J. (1996). Pharmacotherapies for alcohol problems: A review of research with focus on developments since 1991. *Alcoholism, Clinical and Experimental Research, 20,* 859–876.

Littleton, J. (1995). Acamprosate in alcohol dependence: How does it work? *Addiction, 90,* 1179–1188.

Littleton, J., & Little, H. (1994). Current concepts of ethanol dependence. *Addiction, 89,* 1397–1412.

Malcolm, R., Anton, R. F., Randall, C. L., Johnston, A., Brady, K., & Thevos, A. (1992). A placebo-controlled trial of buspirone in anxious inpatient alcoholics. *Alcoholism, Clinical and Experimental Research, 16,* 1007–1013.

Malcolm, R., Ballenger, J. C., Sturgis, E. T., & Anton, R. (1989). Double blind controlled trial comparing carbamazepine to oxazepam treatment of alcohol withdrawal. *American Journal of Psychiatry, 146,* 617–621.

Malec, E., Malec, T., Gagne, M. A., & Dongier, M. (1996). Buspirone in the treatment of alcohol dependence: A placebo-controlled trial. *Alcoholism, Clinical and Experimental Research, 20,* 307–312.

Mason, B. J. (1996). Dosing issues in the pharmacotherapy of alcoholism. *Alcoholism, Clinical and Experimental Research, 20*(Suppl.), 10A–16A.

Mason, B. J., Kocsis, J. H., Ritvo, E. C., & Cutler, R. B. (1996). A double-blind, placebo-controlled trial of desipramine for primary alcohol dependence stratified on the presence or absence of major depression. *Journal of the American Medical Association, 275,* 761–767.

Mason, B. J., Ritvo, E. C., Morgan, R. O., et al. (1994). A double-blind, placebo-controlled pilot study to evaluate the efficacy and safety of oral nalmefene HCl for alcohol dependence. *Alcoholism, Clinical and Experimental Research, 18,* 1162–1167.

McCaul, M. E., Wand, G. S., Sullivan, J., Mumford, G., & Quigley, J. (in press). Betanaltrexol level predicts alcohol relapse [Abstract]. *Alcoholism, Clinical and Experimental Research.*

McGinnis, J. M., & Foege, W. H. (1993). Actual causes of death in the United States. *Journal of the American Medical Association, 270,* 2207–2212.

McGrath, P. J., Nunes, E. V., Stewart, J. W., et al. (1996). Imipramine treatment of alcoholics with major depression: A placebo-controlled clinical trial. *Archives of General Psychiatry, 53,* 232–240.

Monti, P. M., Rohsenow, D. J., Swift, R. M., Abrams, D. B., Colby, S. M., & Mueller, T. L. (in press). Effect of naltrexone on urge to drink during alcohol cue exposure: Preliminary results [Abstract]. *Alcoholism, Clinical and Experimental Research.*

Morse, R. M,, & Flavin, D. K. (1992). Definition of alcoholism. *Journal of the American Medical Association, 268,* 1012–1014.

Mueller, T. I., Stout, R. L., Rudden, S., et al. (1997). A double-blind, placebo-controlled pilot study of carbamazepine for the treatment of alcohol dependence. *Alcoholism, Clinical and Experimental Research, 21,* 86–92.

Nalpas, B., Dabadic, H., Parot, P., & Paccalin, J. (1990). L'acamprosate: De la pharmacologie à la clinique. *Encephale, 16,* 175–179.

Naranjo, C. A., & Bremner, K. E. (1994). Serotonin-altering medications and desire, consumption and effects of alcohol-treatment implications. *EXS, 71,* 209–219.

Naranjo, C. A., Dongier, M., & Bremner, K. E. (1997). Long-acting injectable bromocriptine does not reduce relapse in alcoholics. *Addiction, 92,* 969–978.

Naranjo, C. A., Poulos, C. X., Bremner, K. E., & Lanctot, K. L. (1994). Fluoxetine attenuates alcohol intake and desire to drink. *International Clinical Psychopharmacology, 9,* 163–172.

Naranjo, C. A., Sellers, E. M., Sullivan, J. T., Woodley, D. V., Kadlec, K., & Sykora, K. (1987). The serotonin uptake inhibitor citalopram attenuates ethanol intake. *Clinical Pharmacology and Therapeutics, 41,* 266–274.

Nie, Z., Madamba, S. G., & Siggins, G. R. (1994). Ethanol inhibits glutamatergic neurotransmission in nucleus accumbens neurons by multiple mechanisms. *Journal of Pharmacology and Experimental Therapeutics, 271,* 1566–1573.

O'Malley, S. S., Jaffe, A. J., Chang, G., Schottenfeld, R. S., Meyer, R. E., & Rounsaville, B. (1992). Naltrexone and coping skills therapy for alcohol dependence: A controlled study. *Archives of General Psychiatry, 49,* 881–887.

Peachey, J. E, & Annis, H. (1989). Effectiveness of aversion therapy using disulfiram and related compounds. In K. E. Crow & R. D. Batt (Eds.), *Human metabolism of alcohol. Vol. 1. Pharmacokinetics, medicolegal aspects, and general interests* (pp. 157–169). Boca Raton, FL: CRC Press.

Peachey, J. E., Annis, H. M., Bornstein, E. R., Sykora, K., Maglana, S. M., & Shamai, S. (1989). Calcium carbimide in alcoholism treatment. 1. A placebo-controlled, double-blind clinical trial of short-term efficacy. *British Journal of Addiction, 84,* 877–887.

Peters, D. H., & Faulds, D. (1994). Tiapride: A review of its pharmacology and therapeutic potential in the management of the alcohol dependence syndrome. *Drugs, 47,* 1010–1032.

Poldrugo, F. (1997). Acamprosate treatment in a long-term community-based alcohol rehabilitation programme. *Addiction, 92,* 1537–1546.

Regier, D. A., Farmer, M. E., Rae, D. S., et al. (1990). Comorbidity of mental disorders with alcohol and other drug abuse: Results from the Epidemiologic Catchment Area (ECA) Study. *Journal of the American Medical Association, 264,* 2511–2518.

Rice, D. P. (1993). The economic cost of alcohol abuse and alcohol dependence: 1990. *Alcohol Health and Research World, 17,* 10–11.

Robinson, T. E., & Berridge, K. C. (1993). The neural basis of drug craving: An incentive-sensitization theory of addiction. *Brain Research Reviews, 18,* 247–291.

Rohsenow, D. J., Monti, P. M., Abrams, D. B., et al. (1992). Cue elicited urge to drink and salivation in alcoholics: Relationship to individual differences. *Adv Behav Res Ther, 14,* 195–210.

Salvato, F. R., & Mason, B. J. (1994). Changes in transaminases over the course of a 12-week, double-blind nalmefene trial in a 38-year-old female subject. *Alcoholism, Clinical and Experimental Research, 18,* 1187–1189.

Samson, H. H., & Harris, R. A. (1992). Neurobiology of alcohol abuse. *Trends in Pharmacological Sciences, 13,* 206–211.

Samson, H. H., & Hodge, C. W. (1993). The role of the mesoaccumbens dopamine system in ethanol reinforcement: Studies using the techniques of microinjection and voltammetry. *Alcohol and Alcoholism Supplement, 2,* 469–474.

Sass, H., Soyka, M., Mann, K., & Zieglgansberger, W. (1996). Relapse prevention by acamprosate: Results from a placebo-controlled study on alcohol dependence. *Archives of General Psychiatry, 53,* 673–80. [Erratum. (1996). *Archives of General Psychiatry, 53,* 1097.]

Schuckit, M. A. (1994). Alcohol sensitivity and dependence. *EXS, 71,* 341–348.

Sellers, E. M., Higgins, G. A., & Sobell, M. B. (1992). 5-HT and alcohol abuse. *Trends in Pharmacological Sciences, 13,* 69–75.

Sellers, E. M., Toneatto, T., Romach, M. K., Somer, G. R., Sobell, L. C., & Sobell, M. B. (1994). Clinical efficacy of the 5-HT3 antagonist ondansetron in alcohol abuse and dependence. *Alcoholism, Clinical and Experimental Research, 18,* 879–885.

Shaw, G. K., Waller, S., Majumdar, S. K., Alberts, J. L., Latham, C. J., & Dunn, G. (1994). Tiapride in the prevention of relapse in recently detoxified alcoholics. *British Journal of Psychiatry, 165,* 515–523.

Soyka, M., & Sass, H. (1994). Acamprosate: A new pharmacotherapeutic approach to relapse prevention in alcoholism—preliminary data. *Alcohol and Alcoholism Supplement, 2,* 531–536.

Spanagel, R., Holter, S. M., Allingham, K., Landgraf, R., & Zieglgansberger, W. (1996). Acamprosate and alcohol. I. Effects on alcohol intake following alcohol deprivation in the rat. *European Journal of Pharmacology, 305,* 39–44.

Suzdak, P. D., Schwartz, R. D., Skolnick, P., & Paul, S. M. (1986). Ethanol stimulates gamma-aminobutyric acid receptor-mediated chloride transport in rat brain synaptoneurosomes. *Proceedings of the National Academy of Sciences of the United States of America, 83,* 4071–4075.

Swift, R. M., Whelihan, W., Kuznetsov, O., Buongiorno, G., & Hsuing, H. (1994). Naltrexone-induced alterations in human ethanol intoxication. *American Journal of Psychiatry, 151,* 1463–1467.

Tsai, G., Gastfriend, D. R., & Coyle, J. T. (1995). The glutamatergic basis of human alcoholism. *American Journal of Psychiatry, 152,* 332–340.

Volpicelli, J. R., Alterman, A. I., Hayashida, M., & O'Brien, C. P. (1992). Naltrexone in the treatment of alcohol dependence. *Archives of General Psychiatry, 49,* 876–880.

Volpicelli, J. R., Watson, N. T., King, A. C., Sherman, C. E., & O'Brien, C. P. (1995). Effect of naltrexone on alcohol "high" in alcoholics. *American Journal of Psychiatry, 152,* 613–615.

Volpicelli, J. R., Rhines, K. C., Rhines, J. S., Volpicelli, L. A., Alterman, A. I. & O'Brien, C. P. (1997). Naltrexone and alcohol dependence; role of subject compliance. *Archives of General Psychiatry, 54,* 737–742.

Whitworth, A. B., Fischer, F., Lesch, O. M., et al. (1996). Comparison of acamprosate and placebo in long-term treatment of alcohol dependence. *Lancet, 347,* 1438–1442.

Wise, R. A., & Bozarth, M. A. (1987). A psychomotor stimulant theory of addiction. *Psychological Review, 94,* 469–492.

Zeise, M. L., Kasparov, S., Capogna, M., & Zieglgansberger, W. (1993). Acamprosate (calciumacetylhomotaurinate) decreases postsynaptic potentials in the rat neocortex; possible involvement of excitatory amino acid receptors. *European Journal of Pharmacology, 231,* 47–52.

Chapter 5

Alcoholism Treatment and Medical-Care Costs from Project MATCH

Harold D. Holder, Ph.D.
Ron A. Cisler, Ph.D.
Richard Longabaugh, Ed.D.
Robert L. Stout, Ph.D.
Andrew J. Treno, Ph.D.
Allen Zweben, Ph.D.

INTRODUCTION

Alcoholism treatment effectiveness and costs are contemporary research issues with both health policy and clinical management implications. The problem for medical care administrators today is to determine the most cost-effective treatment approaches for patients, especially with current emphases on cost control and reduction. Cost-effectiveness refers to the effectiveness in clinical outcomes for the least cost (Folland, Goodman, & Stano, 1993; also see discussion by Gold, Siegel, Russell, & Weinstein, 1996). This chapter examines the potential of alcoholism treatment to contribute to health services effects, that is, reduction of total medical-care costs, with special attention to the results achieved by matching patient characteristics to treatment modality.

Three aspects of the potential cost reduction associated with alcoholism treatment can be identified. The first is whether alcoholism treatment, inde-

Research and preparation of this article were supported in part by the National Institute on Alcohol Abuse and Alcoholism grant no. 5 RO1 AA09228 to the Pacific Institute for Research and Evaluation, Chapel Hill, North Carolina.

pendent of treatment modality or setting, can reduce total medical-care utilization and costs. Prior studies of the cost reductions in medical care associated with alcoholism treatment in general are summarized in Jones and Vischi (1979), Holder, Lennox, and Blose (1992), and Holder (1998). A second aspect concerns whether there is differential reduction in total medical-care costs associated with specific treatment modalities, that is, whether specific approaches to recovery have different effects on medical-care utilization and thus costs. The third aspect is whether personal attributes of the patients interact with specific treatment modalities to produce differential changes in total medical-care costs.

This third aspect, with a special relevance to health policy, is concerned with whether patient-matching can yield improved medical-cost outcomes, that is, reduction in total medical-care costs, as discussed initially in Holder, Longabaugh, Miller, and Rubonis (1991). The basic rationale on which such analyses might rest is that if a successful matching of an alcoholic patient to the most appropriate treatment yields improved clinical outcomes, for example, reductions in drinking, then such matching has the potential to stimulate differential medical-care utilization and costs once treatment is begun. In this discussion and throughout this chapter, cost is defined as the actual amount paid to a medical-care service provider, whether it be a client, the government, an insurance company, or other organization. Costs here are, therefore, limited to actual payment for services and do not include other economic considerations. A full cost–benefit study would consider many more outcomes and the economic value of these outcomes. This is well beyond the objectives of this study.

One could argue that patient-matching, broadly construed, is a fundamental theme in health services research. That is, optimum selection of services implies an assessment of an individual's range of problems followed by the selection of a set of services to address those problems (ideally, neither too much nor too little). This matching could be called treatment-service matching. Most patient-treatment matching research has focused on matching for clinical effectiveness. Clinical effectiveness does not, of course, necessarily translate into cost savings for health services, but it may be a necessary precondition for such savings. This chapter reports results from a separate study using patients from two of the MATCH clinical sites, but funded independently of Project MATCH. The project addresses all three of the cost reduction issues described previously by using measures of health utilization and cost collected over a 3-year period after the end of MATCH treatment.

In the United States, Project MATCH itself was a randomized clinical trial treatment study to examine what types of patient–treatment matching improve treatment outcome. Three treatment modalities were used in Project MATCH: cognitive-behavioral therapy (CBT), motivational enhancement therapy (MET) and 12-Step facilitation (TSF). These treatments were examined in relation to 10 primary a priori matching variables (severity of alcohol involvement, cognitive functioning, client conceptual level, gender, meaning seeking, motivational readiness to change, psychiatric severity, social support for drinking versus abstinence, sociopathy, alcohol typology). In addition, 11 secondary a priori matching variables were examined (alcohol dependence, anger, antisocial personality disorder, assertion of autonomy, psychopathology, prior engagement in Alcoholics Anonymous, religiosity, self-efficacy-confidence, self-efficacy-temptation minus confidence, social functioning, and readiness to change). Project MATCH did not include a no-treatment control group, as its purpose was to examine the relative clinical effectiveness of three specific treatment modalities allowing for any interactions with the personal attributes of the client.

In sum, of the 10 primary matching variables examined, only two statistically significant matching effects were found: psychiatric severity and network support for drinking (Project MATCH Research Group, 1997a, 1998a). More specifically, in the 1-year posttreatment period, outpatients low in psychiatric severity had significantly greater percentage of abstinent days after TSF than after CBT (Project MATCH Research Group, 1997a). Also, patients with a social network supportive of drinking had more percentage days abstinent and fewer drinks per drinking day with TSF than with MET; this latter finding emerged only at the 3-year follow-up (Project MATCH Research Group, 1998a). Of the 11 secondary matching variables examined, also only two statistically significant matching effects were found: anger and alcohol dependence (Project MATCH Research Group, 1997b). As hypothesized, those outpatients receiving MET who were high in anger at intake were abstinent more often and drank less when they did drink at 1 and 3 years follow-up than CBT clients. Also consistent with hypothesized effects, aftercare patients who were low in dependence at intake had more abstinent days at follow-up with CBT than with TSF; conversely, aftercare patients who were high in dependence at intake had better drinking outcomes with TSF than with CBT at follow-up. The three treatments did not differ from one another in producing clinically significant differences in the two primary drinking outcomes, percentage of days abstinent and drinks per drinking day (Project MATCH Research Group, 1997a, 1997b, 1998a).

In terms of the relative costs of replicating these three treatments in typical clinical settings, Cisler, Holder, Longabaugh, Stout, and Zweben (1998) estimated that the average per-patient costs for treatment ranged from $359 for MET to $407 for TSF to $433 for CBT. Estimates were calculated on actual treatment utilization data (average utilization of therapy sessions was 8.14, 3.19, and 7.40 for CBT, MET, and TSF, respectively); estimated per-session therapists costs; and costs for reading materials, assessment procedures, and laboratory procedures. All cost figures were derived from estimates provided by senior investigators at each of the nine Project MATCH sites. In terms of average costs, MET was $48 less than TSF (12% less) and $74 less than CBT (17% less). When utilization of these treatments, however, were at their highest (i.e., 10.36, 3.58, and 9.37 sessions for CBT, MET, and TSF, respectively), estimated per-patient costs ranged from $512 for MET to $750 for TSF to $788 for CBT: MET cost $238 less than TSF (32% less) and $276 less than CBT (35% less). For the present study, these estimated treatment cost differentials are included in equations examining treatment and posttreatment utilization and costs of alcoholism treatment and other medical and behavioral health services.

The present study attempts to extend our understanding of the effects of patient–treatment matching on total medical-care cost. Like Project MATCH, this study did not include a no-treatment control group, and the inferences are limited to the comparisons across and among the three treatment modalities. No comparison to no treatment is possible with this design. Project MATCH has been criticized previously for relying mainly on measures of alcohol consumption and consumption-related consequences in determining the value of MATCH treatment (cf. Commentaries published in *Addiction*, 1999). Failure to include broader measures of outcome dealing with quality of life and economic issues has raised questions about the utility of MATCH findings to "real world" treatment settings by Drummond (1999). Without considering the economic aspects of treatment, payers of alcohol treatment services may be unable to decide whether effective MATCH treatments are worth the additional costs of training and supervising therapists in these modalities (Godfrey, 1999).

This chapter explores the three aspects of potential reductions in medical costs as described previously: (a) whether medical-care costs declined after alcoholism treatment is initiated across all modalities in Project MATCH; (b) whether there are differences across the three treatment modalities utilized in this project, considering posttreatment initiation medical costs; and (c) whether there are interactional effects of patient matching on posttreatment initiation medical-care costs. The first two analyses provide an essential basis for the third consideration, that is, the effects of patient-matching. It should be noted that this is the only known study in which both treatment main effects and matching are tested for their effects on posttreatment medical-care costs under a condition of random assignment to treatment. In addition, no prior studies have examined medical-care costs in relation to TSF. Project MATCH was the first randomized controlled clinical trial that evaluated the clinical effectiveness of TSF. Given the widespread utilization of TSF, having medical-care cost data on this modality was expected to be particularly useful to policy makers in the alcoholism treatment field.

METHODS

Subjects and Settings

Subjects were 279 of 430 Project MATCH participants at two of the nine MATCH Clinical Research Units (i.e., Providence, RI and Milwaukee, WI), representing about 65% of the individuals treated at these sites. These individuals agreed to be part of the present study that entailed an extended follow-up period of 2 years beyond the 1 year follow-up of Project MATCH. As part of their involvement in this study, subjects also agreed to have their insurance and medical records reviewed for analyses of costs. Subjects were drawn from two distinct aftercare settings in Providence, Rhode Island and from both a private, for-profit outpatient clinic and various inpatient settings in Milwaukee, Wisconsin.

Table 5.1 summarizes analyses conducted to examine potential differences between subjects who were recruited and agreed to participate ($n = 279$) and those who were recruited but did not participate in the cost study ($n = 151$). Participants differed from nonparticipants only with respect to gender: a

TABLE 5.1. Sociodemographic and Pretreatment Severity Comparisons of Cost-Study Participants ($n = 279$) and Nonparticipants ($n = 151$)

Characteristic	Participants ($n = 279$)	Sample Nonparticipants ($n = 151$)	Statistic
Age (mean ± SD)	40.11 ± 11.72	41.59 ± 11.85	$F = 1.58$
Gender (%)			
Female	35%	24%	$\chi^2 = 5.66*$
Male	65%	76%	
Ethnicity (%)			
White	92%	91%	$\chi^2 = 1.53$
Black	6%	5%	
Hispanic	1%	3%	
Other	1%	1%	
Years of formal education (mean ± SD)	13.20 ± 2.09	13.43 ± 2.40	$F = 1.11$
Relationship status (%)			
Couple	36%	44%	$\chi^2 = 2.57$
Single	64%	56%	
Employment status (%)			
Employed	49%	58%	$\chi^2 = 2.81$
Not employed	51%	42%	
Prior alcohol treatment (%)			
Yes	58%	58%	$F = 0.01$
No	42%	42%	
Alcohol dependence symptoms[a] (mean ± SD)	6.15 ± 2.09	6.34 ± 2.10	$F = 0.80$
ASI psychiatric severity[b] (mean ± SD)	0.22 ± 0.21	0.22 ± 0.22	$F = 0.01$

*$p<0.05$; **$p<0.01$; ***$p<0.001$.
[a]Measured by SCID for the 90-day period prior to enrollment; symptom counts range from 1 to 9.
[b]Composite score derived from the Addiction Severity Index; higher score indicates higher severity.

greater proportion of participants were female (35%) than those who refused to participate in the present cost study (24%). Participants and nonparticipants were similar statistically with respect to age, ethnicity, education, relationship status, employment status, prior alcohol treatment, alcohol dependence symptoms, and psychiatric symptom severity.

Individuals refused to participate for a number of reasons, including: 74 who initially agreed to participate but were unable or unwilling to sign a second (and in some cases a third) modified consent-to-release-data form required by changes in state laws; 37 who agreed to participate and signed consent forms but the available data were inadequate for analysis; 20 who could not be located during follow-up; 10 who died during follow-up; 7 who refused to participate; and 3 who had moved from the area from where they were recruited.

Additional analyses were conducted to examine potential differences between Project MATCH subjects who were recruited and participated in the cost study ($n = 279$) and the larger MATCH patient population (consisting of subjects who were not recruited or who were recruited but did not agree to participate in the cost study ($n = 1,447$). Briefly, the present cost-study sample and the rest of the Project MATCH sample were similar with respect to age, years of formal education, relationship status (couple or single), employment status (employed, unemployed), alcohol dependence symptoms, and psychiatric symptoms. The two samples differed statistically, however, on gender, ethnicity, and history of alcohol treatment. The present cost-study participants consisted of proportionately more females (35%) and fewer ethnic minorities (8%) and were more likely to have a history of alcohol treatment (58%) than the other Project MATCH participants (22%, 22%, and 49%, respectively). The sample from the two sites was not intended to be representative of all Project MATCH sites and thus these results could be generalized to these other sites and to other clinical settings only with considerable caution.

Study Variables

For cost analyses, three dependent variables were developed: (a) inpatient care costs, (b) outpatient care costs, and (c) total medical costs. We did not analyze emergency room (ER) costs separately, as the use of the ER by this clinical population was low. We coded the ER costs in with the outpatient costs with no loss of detail. Whereas the original design for data collection was to focus on insurance companies and medical archives as data sources, the U.S. medical-care system changed dramatically during the early stages of the project. Specifically, the system that emerged was characterized by multiple insurers, health maintenance organizations, managed-care providers, and self-insurers. Thus, cost and utilization data were captured through a triangulated system that involved collection of data from three primary sources: (a) hospitals, (b) insurance companies, and (c) providers. Respondents were asked at approximately 90-day intervals to complete health insurance/health-provider forms at the Wisconsin and Rhode Island sites. These forms provided self-reports of medical services received and were used primarily to locate service providers. All providers, insurance companies, and hospitals were contacted with rigorous follow-up and asked to provide cost and utilization data for all contacts with that patient. This procedure permitted capture of data that may have been unreported by the quarterly self-report. It is important to note here that we are considering hospital charges as a surrogate measure for medical-care costs. Obviously, this underestimates total costs, which include individual level (e.g., lost income) and societal level (e.g., lost productivity) costs.

All medical-care data collected were coded and used to create a raw dataset. These data could be single procedures up to full hospitalization costs. Duplicate data were removed, as were all pharmacy, dental, and residence-only cost data. Data were then segregated into inpatient versus outpatient. ER data were coded as inpatient if they immediately preceded a hospitalization or detox event, but otherwise were considered as outpatient. Inpatient data were then aggregated to the event level subsuming any concurrent outpatient charges (e.g., pathology laboratory, surgeon's fees, etc.). The result was an events dataset divided into inpatient and outpatient events of utilization and costs.

When cost data were lacking or incomplete, estimates were derived based upon type of event, length of stay, and DRG or ICD-9 codes. Forty-six percent of reported events did not initially have associated costs based on the data provided to the project and required estimation. American Hospital Association Statistics were used to obtain hospital-cost expense estimates. Specifically, we used hospital total expenses adjusted per inpatient day for community hospitals for each state (Wisconsin and Rhode Island) for each year. The Center for Health Care Evaluation, Department of Veterans Affairs of Stanford University provided us with the average cost per day for six types of inpatient events for each year, including inpatient substance abuse or psychiatric unit, inpatient medical, inpatient surgical, inpatient intermediate care, nursing home care, and domiciliary care. When all medical-care events had an associated cost (in current dollars), costs were converted to constant 1982–1984 dollars using the CPI-U for hospital and related services (SE57) for inpatient events, and the CPI-U for professional medical services (SE56) for outpatient events, and adjusted for the appropriate region (North Central for Wisconsin and North East for Rhode Island). Finally, data were aggregated for each patient for inpatient and for outpatient costs per 30-day period since joining the MATCH project. Events that fell into more than one period were prorated uniformly and the mean cost per day allocated to the appropriate period. The highest event cost per period was assigned an upper value of $7,500, or two standard deviations from the mean. Except for the sorting for missing cost and CPI-U values, inpatient and outpatient data were treated similarly. Further, self-reported events that were not represented in the collected data were entered and treated as collected data with missing cost information. The self-reported events were not merged with collected data, but were prepared on parallel tracks so they could be included or excluded more readily.

Alcoholism treatment costs for the three Project MATCH treatment modalities were calculated by multiplying the number of sessions of MATCH treatment each subject had in each month by the mean estimated replication cost for that treatment (Cisler et al., 1998). Average costs associated with the dosage and other treatment protocol differences (Cisler et al., 1998) were entered into cost analyses as a constant to control for their potential differential effects. The final sample sizes for each MATCH treatment modality were: CBT, 89; MET, 94; and TSF, 96.

Project MATCH measured alcohol consumption by quantity and frequency of alcohol consumption on a daily and weekly basis as a part of overall evaluation. Subjects reported the number of standard ethanol content drinks, equaling 0.5 oz (15 ml) of alcohol consumed, and the time period in which they were consumed. During Project MATCH, drinking was assessed roughly once every 3 months beginning at intake, immediately following 3 months of treatment, and at 3-month intervals over a 12-month posttreatment follow-up period, totaling about 540 continuous days. For the present cost study, subjects were interviewed every 6 months for an additional 2 years posttreatment, totaling about 1,260 continuous days. Two primary dependent measures were used to measure alcohol consumption: percentage days abstinent (PDA), providing a measure of drinking frequency; and drinks per drinking day (DDD), providing a measure of drinking severity (Babor et al., 1994; Project MATCH Research Group, 1997a).

This chapter presents the results from three sets of research questions. The statistical analyses for each question are unique to that question and the Results section for the convenience of the reader.

RESULTS

Overall Treatment and Individual Modality Effects on Medical Costs

The first question was whether Project MATCH treatments individually reduced medical costs in the aggregate. Time-series analyses involving pre- and postalcoholism treatment initiation periods (73 months in total composed of 36 months in either direction plus 1 month of treatment initiation). Only inpatient costs were used. Outpatient costs for the pretreatment period were not sufficiently reliable to be used in the time-series analyses. Inpatient costs were by far the largest percentage of total costs and a good surrogate for total costs. Prior studies of potential medical cost reduction have found that inpatient costs account for most of total medical costs and are the most affected by alcoholism treatment (Holder & Blose, 1992; Holder, 1998). Four time-series were

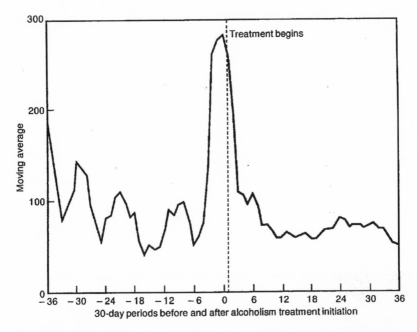

FIGURE 5.1. Monthly average inpatient cost per patient, Project MATCH (USA)—Wisconsin and Rhode Island sites only in 1982–1984 constant dollars.

created: one for all subjects and one for each of the three treatment protocols. The time-series were conducted on average inpatient cost in constant 1982–1984 U.S. dollars per 30-day period relative to program intake. Figure 5.1 presents these costs for 3 years prior to and 3 years posttreatment with a 30-day period moving average. Visual inspection suggests that inpatient costs declined in the posttreatment period. Additionally, there appeared to be a decline in the variance of these estimates over time and between treatments (Box & Jenkins, 1976).

As a statistical test of observed-over-time differences, a series of autoregressive interrupted moving average (ARIMA) models were estimated (Box & Jenkins, 1976). This procedure involves the examination of autocorrelation and partial autocorrelation patterns within the time-series, the estimation of models incorporating parameters adjusting for these patterns, and analysis of residuals for remaining autocorrelation. Data were differenced and an AR1 parameter included to account for diagnosed autocorrelation. The results from the four analyses, overall and three treatment-specific, are presented in Table 5.2. Significant differences overall and for each treatment type for the posttreatment period indicate a decline in average per-patient cost in the post-initiation-of-treatment period. The pre- and posttreatment monthly

TABLE 5.2. Comparison of Posttreatment Costs to Pretreatment
Costs, Time Series (ARIMA) Modeling

	Beta	T-ratio	p-value
CBT			
Constant	6.009	0.473	0.638
AR1*	−0.357	_3.012	0.004
Postintervention	−409.483	−2.982	0.004
MET			
Constant	5.316	0.399	0.691
AR1*	−0.036	−0.291	0.772
Postintervention	−777.026	−6.640	<0.000
TSF			
Constant	1.790	0.210	0.834
AR1*	−0.182	−1.536	0.129
Postintervention	−352.276	−4.201	<0.000
Overall			
Constant	5.676	0.631	0.530
AR1*	0.088	0.656	0.514
Postintervention	−603.068	−8.681	<0.000

*AR1 = autoregressive component with $\log_1$.

means were: overall, $653 versus $186; CBT, $913 versus $328; MET, $827 versus $176; and TSF, $503 versus $225. Analysis of residuals indicated little, if any, remaining autocorrelation. The analyses suggest that alcoholism treatment is associated with a reduction in total medical-care costs across all MATCH treatment modalities and across individual treatment modalities.

Main Effects and Costs

Going beyond the question of whether alcoholism treatment in the aggregate is associated with medical-care cost reduction, the second question can be asked: Is variability in posttreatment reduction in medical-care costs associated with the kind of clinical intervention implemented? This question addressed whether the three different treatment modalities are associated with differences in overall medical-care costs. An earlier review of cost-effectiveness of alcohol treatments (Holder et al., 1991) concluded that: (a) some alcohol treatments were more effective than others, (b) some treatments were less costly to implement than were others, and (c) some treatments were both more effective and less costly to implement than others. The general conclusion was that, in order to evaluate the medical-care cost reduction, one could not simply compare any alcohol treatment with no intervention: it was necessary to compare specifically designated treatments under condition of random assignment (Holder et al., 1991).

The MATCH study compared three treatments. Two were already established as clinically effective: CBT and motivational interviewing (Miller et al., 1995). CBT and brief motivational counseling (Holder et al., 1991) differed in their estimated cost of implementation, with motivationally based brief interventions in the least costly category and CBT in the next level of cost. The third MATCH treatment, TSF, implemented a version of a widely used treatment, the Minnesota Model, that did not have sufficient evidence to judge either its effectiveness or costs (Holder et al., 1991).

MATCH found these three treatments not to differ appreciably in their effectiveness in reducing drinking. The present study examines whether they differ in their medical costs. While the earlier work of the present research group (Cisler et al., 1998) established that MET was less costly to deliver than CBT or TSF, the question of whether MET results in overall medical-cost savings needs to be answered. It could be that these initial cost savings from MET are dwarfed by subsequent medical costs that result from their receiving insufficient alcohol treatment from MET.

Medical-care costs for hospitalization (by far the greatest cost) and outpatient costs and, thus, total costs following treatment initiation, were sufficiently reliable to permit tests of main effects as well as patient matching. Estimated costs for MATCH treatment were also included in these analyses. Medical-care costs after alcoholism treatment begin a steeply declining time course, as shown in Figure 5.1. To analyze treatment and matching effects, we employed latent growth analysis methods (Bryk & Raudenbush, 1992; Carbonari, Wirtz, Muenz, & Stout, 1994). These models used both a linear time trend term to represent any secular trend in medical costs posttreatment and an exponentially declining time term to model the rapidly declining portion of the utilization curve, or a "ramp-down" term.

The main effects for the matching variables, treatment, and other covariates were determined as follows. In all analyses we covaried for baseline medical-care costs because health conditions associated with high costs can persist from the baseline period into the outcome period. Because of rapid changes in medical-care utilization in the months just prior to treatment (Holder et al., 1992), we computed baseline medical costs for two periods: (a) a ramp-up baseline period including the 3 months immediately before treatment and (b) a longer term baseline period that included the 9 months preceding the ramp-up period. Mean costs were computed using a natural log transformation to reduce skewness for both periods. Since medical care use is influenced by a number of background variables including age, gender, and ethnicity, these variables were included as a priori covariates. To determine treatment effects, we also covaried baseline indicators of addictions severity (baseline scores for percentage of days abstinent and drinks per drinking day, as well as SCID symptom count). Since site differences were found in Project MATCH (Project MATCH Research Group, 1997a), we also covaried for site effects, including both site main effects and site by treatment interactions (in our study, there were four clinical sites as defined in the MATCH analyses). We removed from our models any of these covariates that did not have statistically significant effects on cost outcome. The remaining basic covariates were used in analyses for the main effects for treatment, and also the patient–treatment matching analyses.

One would expect that drinking would be highly associated with medi-cal-care utilization and, therefore, costs based upon studies of heavy drinkers via hospital admissions. Therefore, we hypothesized that we would find a direct association between drinking and medical-care costs in this analysis. Because of the skewness of the data, simple Spearman correlations were used to deter-mine the association between drinking at one point in time and medical costs at the same point in time. As shown in Table 5.3, the associations are not high. For example, 1 year after treatment, the correlations are all nonsignificant be-tween 0.058 (percentage days abstinent) and 0.024 (drinks per drinking day).

Analyses of patient–treatment matching were performed by adding new terms to the main effects analyses. In the matching analyses, the main effect of the matching variable was included as a term in the model, as well as the matching variable by treatment interaction. The basic covariates were also included as described above. The main effects for the matching variables were determined during the course of the patient–treatment matching analyses.

While there is a dramatic decrease in medical costs immediately follow-ing MATCH treatment, as signaled by a strongly significant ramp-down term ($F(1,188) = 109.23$, $p < 0.0001$), there is also a statistically significant linear trend ($F(1,188) = 26.63$, $p < 0.0001$), indicating a long-term upward trend in medical costs, estimated to be $13 per month on average. The main effects of the basic baseline covariates are shown in Table 5.3. The beta coefficients reported in Table 5.4 indicate the amount of increase in monthly posttreatment costs per unit increase in the covariate. For example, because baseline medical costs were $\log_{10}$ transformed, the beta value of 114 indicates that for every tenfold increase in baseline costs, follow-up costs increased by $114 per month. Statistically significant site main effects and site by linear time interactions

TABLE 5.3. Effect of Covariates on Posttreatment Medical-Care Costs

Effect	p-value	Regression coefficient (SE)
Mean monthly cost, long-term BL ($\log_{10}$)	0.0004	+ 113.7 (31.6)
Age (years)	0.0001	+ 6.9 (1.6)
SCID symptom count, BL	0.0003	+ 34.4 (9.4)
Percentage of days abstinent, BL	0.0003	+ 2.3 (0.6)
Clinical research unit	0.0256	See text
Clinical research unit by linear time interaction	0.0240	See text

TABLE 5. 4. Clinical Effectiveness and Cost Savings of MATCH Treatments
(Based on Total Costs, Years 1–3)

Patient characteristic	Level	Comparison of clinical effectiveness	**Cost savings per year	Total cost savings over 3 years
Alcohol dependence	High	TSF < CBT*	$293 TSF↑	$879
	Low	CBT > TSF*	$271 CBT↑	$813
Psychiatric severity	High	CBT = MET	$996 CBT↑	$2,988
	Low	MET = CBT	$1,305 MET↑	$3,915
Network support for drinking	High	CBT = MET	$614 CBT↑	$1,842
	Low	MET = CBT	$1,457 MET↑	$4,371

*MATCH after-care sites, only (Project MATCH Research Group, 1998b). **Based on annualized costs dichotomized over 3-year period. ↑ indicates the treatment that is more likely to produce medical-care cost savings.

were detected. The site differences are likely to be due to regional differences in medical costs, and also to baseline differences in the subject samples on covariates not included in these analyses. As predictors of follow-up costs, higher prior medical-care costs and age were associated with elevated post-treatment medical care costs, as expected. Two clinical variables were found to predict costs. Higher values for SCID symptom count at treatment intake were found to be associated with higher costs. For percentage of days abstinent, we found that those subjects who displayed more abstinence at baseline also exhibited *higher* posttreatment medical care costs. No matching variables were found to have statistically significant main effects after the standard covariates were included in the model. Three matching variables (gender, cognitive impairment, and social support for drinking) were observed to have main effects if baseline costs, age, and baseline alcohol variables were omitted from the model.

There were no statistically significant main effects for the Project MATCH treatments ($F(2,188) = 2.06$, $p = 0.1303$). The mean estimated monthly post-treatment costs for the three conditions ranged from a low of $254 for MET subjects to a high of $315 for CBT and $310 for TSF.

The two clinical variables were found to predict costs, however, and presented something of a paradox. The fact that higher values for SCID symptom count at treatment intake were found to be associated with higher costs is consistent with the belief that higher clinical severity should be associated with higher costs. However, it was surprising to find that those cases less severe on the percentage of days abstinent measure tended to have higher costs.

The lack of treatment main effects on medical costs is understandable in the context of the limited differences in the clinical outcomes found in Project MATCH (Project MATCH Research Group, 1997a, 1997b). The ranking of the treatments by their medical costs, however, is of substantive importance given the nature of the MET treatment. MET was included in Project MATCH as a brief alternative to the more traditional and intensive CBT and TSF. It was expected that should clinical outcomes for MET cases be comparable to those for the other treatments, then MET might be found to be an attractive treatment on cost-effectiveness grounds. Indeed, our analyses of Project MATCH treatment costs indicate that MET does have a cost advantage relative to the other treatments (Cisler et al., 1998). This advantage in initial treatment cost, however, might have been undermined if MET subjects experienced higher post-MATCH medical costs. Our data do not provide any evidence to support higher medical costs for MET cases; indeed, MET cases have the lowest post-MATCH costs. Thus, our data provide further support for the cost-effectiveness of MET treatment relative to CBT and TSF.

Matching Effects and Costs

A third question for this study was posed by Holder et al. (1991): Given that some treatment modalities might be more cost-effective than others for the average patient, could some treatments be matched to patient characteristics to improve the effectiveness of the treatment for such patients? This question was addressed in the present study for the first time by examining the potential interaction of patient variables with treatment modalities and medical costs.

Prior findings with the total Project MATCH study population indicated that when drinking was the focus of concern, matching effects were infrequent and modest. However, given the small correlations between the primary drinking measures and medical-care costs (reported above), matching effects on medical-care costs may be independent of matching effects on drinking. Above, we reported that treatment effects on medical-care costs were independent of matching variables. Here we report the moderating effects of some of these patient variables on main treatment effects.

When drinking was considered the primary dependent variable, we identified matching effects involving four patient variables: alcohol dependence, psychiatric severity, anger, and network support for drinking. When medical-care costs are considered, three of these same four matching variables appear to be implicated in modest matching effects (patient anger being the fourth).

There is a consistency in results across these three variables, in that matching effects are observed for inpatient and total costs across the 3-year period, whereas outpatient costs (the cost measure least sensitive to alcoholism treatment) are unaffected.

Alcohol Dependence

First, identical to the matching effect found with drinking, alcohol dependence interacts with CBT versus TSF treatment assignment to effect inpatient (CBT

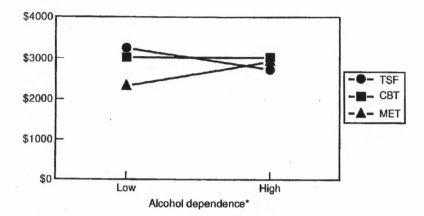

FIGURE 5.2. Total costs, years 1–3, alcohol dependence. For purposes of displaying the results, the figure is based on the means of groups based on a median split into "high" and low." The statistical test of matching efforts was based on a comparison of the slopes of the three treatment groups.

vs. TSF, $t = 2.16$, $p < 0.03$) and total ($t = 2.11$ $p < 0.03$) medical-care costs (see Figure 5.2). Irrespective of variability in alcohol dependence, the treatment costs of CBT are invariant, whereas TSF patients with low dependence incur more medical-care costs, while those with high dependence incur fewer medical-care costs. The result is that patients with low dependence have lower medical-care costs when treated with CBT than TSF, while patients with high dependence have lower medical-care costs when treated with TSF.

Also of interest, particularly in the context of the tendency toward better overall cost-effectiveness of MET at low levels of alcohol dependence, MET patients have costs lower than both CBT and TSF, but at high levels of dependence, the three groups are indistinguishable.

Psychiatric Severity

Assignment to CBT interacts with patient psychiatric severity, as expected. As psychiatric severity increases, patients treated in CBT have lower inpatient and total costs relative to MET patients ($t = -2.16$, $p < 0.03$ inpatient costs, $t = -2.11$, $p < 0.03$ total costs) (see Figure 5.3). The hypothesis was that CBT would be more effective than MET in treating patients with higher levels of psychiatric severity because of CBT's focus on teaching intrapersonal skills for dealing with high-risk situations, such as those involving negative affect. Because MET assumes that the patient already has the psychological and social resources for coping with his/her alcohol problem, providing only four treatment sessions, it was hypothesized that patients with greater psychiatric severity would be mismatched to MET (Project MATCH Research Group,

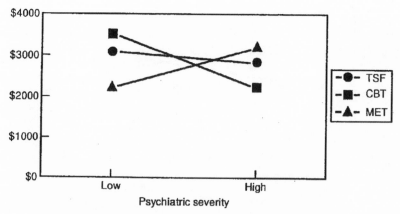

FIGURE 5.3. Total costs, years 1–3, psychiatric severity.

1997a). In Figure 5.3, a review of the slopes for the two treatments as a function of psychiatric severity supports these differential effects. As Addiction Severity Index (ASI) severity increases, inpatient and total costs of CBT patients diminish, whereas the opposite appears to be true for MET patients, for whom costs increase increasing with increased psychiatric severity.

Network Support for Drinking

Network support for drinking also interacts with CBT versus MET treatment assignment (see Figure 5.4). For patients with social networks unsupportive of drinking, MET patients incur less inpatient and total treatment costs than do CBT patients. However, for patients with networks more supportive of drinking, CBT patients have fewer costs than MET patients (CBT vs. MET slopes, inpatient costs, $t = -0.210$, $p < 0.036$; total costs, $t = -0.243$, $p < 0.015$). Fur-

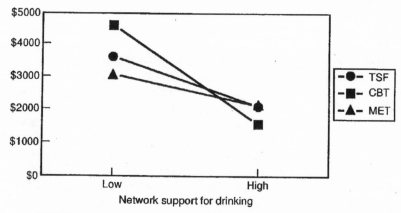

FIGURE 5.4. Total costs, years 1–3, network support for drinking.

thermore, the differences in total medical-care costs for those matched versus mismatched are not trivial: for those low in network support for drinking, assignment to MET versus CBT saves $1,457; for those with networks supportive of drinking assignment to CBT rather than MET saves $614.

Clinical Effectiveness and Medical Care Costs of MATCH Treatments

A major aim of the present study was to determine whether there is a differential reduction in cost savings and level of improvement across different patient-treatment matching contrasts. MATCH patients were categorized as high or low on variables found to have matching effects (i.e., alcohol dependence, psychiatric severity, network support) and compared on both measures of clinical effectiveness (i.e., drinking improvement) and medical-cost savings over a 3-year period. Data on clinical effectiveness were derived from Project MATCH 3-year drinking outcomes (Project MATCH, 1998a). For example, CBT patients high on psychiatric severity were compared to their MET counterparts in terms of drinking improvement and the amount of cost savings after exposure to these different treatment modalities.

Table 5.4 summarizes the findings on clinical effectiveness and medical-care cost saving. TSF demonstrates a healthcare cost-savings advantage over CBT for individuals high on alcohol dependence, while CBT performs similarly among individuals low on alcohol dependence. Thus, drinking improvement found among highly dependent TSF patients and low-dependent CBT patients eventually translates into cost savings in healthcare services for these patient groups (see Table 5.4). One caution, despite the fact that TSF showed a cost-savings advantage over CBT for highly dependent patients, and CBT over TSF for low-dependent patients, MET was still found to have the greatest potential for healthcare cost savings. It was not the most clinically effective of the three MATCH treatment modalities either for patients with low dependence (CBT was) or high dependence (TSF was).

CBT shows evidence of a healthcare cost-savings advantage over MET for individuals high on psychiatric severity, while MET performs better than CBT for individuals low on this dimension. Similarly, CBT demonstrates a cost-savings advantage over MET for individuals whose networks are supportive of the drinking, while the opposite is the case for individuals whose networks are not supportive of drinking: MET shows a considerable cost-savings advantage over CBT with the latter group.

DISCUSSION

The matching results for cost outcomes indicate that the overall superiority of MET over the other more intensive treatments is apparent only for those patients who have good prognostic characteristics on alcohol dependence, psychiatric severity, and/or network support for drinking. MET has a clear advantage over the other two MATCH treatments with patients having these good prognostic characteristics. The MET approach encourages patients to utilize their own inner resources to combat alcohol problems, and patients who are likely to succeed in their change plans (i.e., good prognostic patients) might be more likely to draw upon and effectively use their own capabilities to do so. Thus, for these good prognostic patients, 3 to 4 sessions of MET may be sufficient to sustain their improvement and/or prevent them from acquiring additional services.

These findings are in marked contrast to the potential health-cost savings for patients with poor prognostic indicators on psychiatric severity, network support for drinking, and alcohol dependence. For patients with high psychiatric severity and those who have networks highly supportive of drinking, CBT is a better cost-savings alternative than MET. As shown earlier, at low levels of severity, MET has the best cost-savings return, but this cost advantage decreases as severity increases. While MET may be as effective in reducing drinking for these poor prognostic patients, in the long term it costs more for the MET patient to achieve this effect than for the CBT patient (see Table 5.4). With poor prognostic patients, CBT may help them obtain relevant skills to ward off some negative effects of excessive drinking without substantially effecting the drinking, at least in the short term. It is conceivable then, that CBT serves as a mechanism to reduce the negative consequences of drinking for this patient group, which eventually translates into a cost advantage for this treatment modality.

It is possible that the matching findings on medical-care costs could have been obtained by chance alone, since only 3 of the hypothesized 21 matching variables were implicated. We think this is unlikely. First, the matching variables that were observed to affect health-cost outcomes were 3 of the 4 also observed in the main MATCH trial to affect drinking outcomes. In addition, all the 17 matching variables that failed to demonstrate matching effects in Project MATCH on drinking outcomes also failed to demonstrate matching effects on cost outcomes. Thus, it would seem that those patient factors that affected healthcare costs also affected drinking, while those that did not affect cost also did not affect drinking. If costs and drinking were closely related to one another, this coincidence could be attributed to lack of independence between cost and drinking outcomes. However, the lack of correlation between drinking and healthcare costs suggests this not to be the case. The more likely alternative, then, is that these three variables are valid indicators for matching.

All three of the matching effects observed were hypothesized a priori. Of interest, however, the treatment contrasts showing greatest matching effects when health cost is the dependent variable are different from those observed to have the greatest effects on drinking outcomes. For example, individuals whose networks are supportive of drinking fared better in TSF than in MET in relation to drinking while this same group had lower posttreatment healthcare costs when assigned to CBT than to MET. That all observed matching effects were hypothesized a priori strengthens their credibility.

An important context for understanding these effects was the shared belief among the Project MATCH Research Group that MET would provide insufficient treatment for the more severely dysfunctional patients. Consequently, seven of the matching hypotheses involved contrasts of MET with one and/or the other of the two more intensive treatments, CBT and TSF (Project MATCH Research Group, 1997a, 1997b). Contrary to expectations, the pattern of results led the MATCH researchers to conclude that MET was just as effective in reducing drinking of more severely dysfunctional patients than the more intensive treatments (Project MATCH Research Group, 1997a). Results from the present cost analyses suggest that the original thinking underlying the a priori hypotheses (as opposed to the post hoc interpretation) may not have been totally in error.

Study Limitations

The current study is not without its limitations, and future research is encouraged to take these into account. First, it must be noted that the original design of Project MATCH did not employ a no-treatment control group. Therefore, it cannot be inferred that the observed differences in healthcare costs were due to the impact of the study treatments. Second, a complex system of data collection from multiple sources including hospitals and individual providers was implemented. In a time of rapid changes in the medical-care system in the United States, some providers either refused to provide data or were unable to do so, particularly small providers of outpatient services. Fortunately, for the validity of the study, the lion's share of total healthcare costs was accounted for by inpatient services, for which we were able to obtain exact costs or valid estimates. Third, missing cost estimates for self-report data could not be matched to verified costs. Thus, imputed costs had to be estimated based upon averages for type of event. We found no reason to believe that any systematic biases were present in health event reporting. Fourth, this is a smaller group of clients from only two MATCH treatment sites. As such, these results cannot be generalized to other sites. Certainly, as this is a first study of its type, replication in other locations and with a larger study population is desired.

CONCLUSIONS AND RECOMMENDATIONS

The present findings suggest that there may be some real cost advantages in triaging alcohol patients to specialized treatments based, at least, on some of the attributes studied and treatments offered in Project MATCH. From a policy standpoint, consideration should be given to employing MET with good prognostic patients (i.e., low psychiatric severity and low network support for drinking), particularly in settings where the costs of the alternative approaches are high, and it is doubtful whether they would produce outcomes beyond those already offered in MET with this population. For patients high in psychiatric severity and/or whose networks are supportive of drinking, CBT offers significant cost savings when compared to MET. Thus, it would be reasonable to steer these poor prognostic patients to CBT, especially in settings where available treatments have not been shown to be advantageous in terms of efficacy (e.g., MET) over this particular modality with this patient group. For patients high on alcohol dependence, TSF produces greater cost savings than CBT. TSF has also demonstrated greater improvement in drinking behavior than CBT with these poor prognostic patients (Project MATCH Research Group, 1998). Thus, from a cost-savings viewpoint, TSF should be given priority over CBT in selecting treatment options for highly dependent patients, while CBT should be given priority for low-dependent patients. Finally, it should be noted that the healthcare cost savings resulting from MATCH treatments were not as high for poor prognostic patients compared to good prognostic patients.

Future Research

From the perspective of policy makers, there still remains the concern of how to maximize the clinical effectiveness of alcoholism treatment while reducing healthcare costs. The present study revealed that drinking improvement does not necessarily translate into reduced healthcare costs for certain patient groups. Therefore, the ongoing challenge for investigators is to develop a repertoire of interventions geared to addressing the diverse capacities and needs of alcohol patients and at the same time show significant healthcare cost savings. Such studies are particularly relevant to providers and payers who need to be concerned about both clinical and economic aspects of alcoholism treatment.

Finally, the present cost study has shed new light on the importance of patient–treatment matching in the alcoholism treatment field. These findings can be utilized to formulate new policy guidelines for patient–treatment matching. It is hoped that the study can serve as a model to alcohol researchers interested in adding a cost component to their research designs and can stimulate them to do so. This would help move the field further along in understanding the interface between healthcare costs and treatment effectiveness.

REFERENCES

Babor, T. F., Longabaugh, R., Zweben, A., Fuller, R. K., Stout, R. L., Anton, R. F., & Randall, C. L. (1994). Issues in the definition and measurement of drinking outcomes in alcoholism treatment research, *Journal of Studies on Alcohol, Suppl. 12,* 101–111.

Bryk, A. S., & Raudenbush, S. W. (1992). *Hierarchical linear models.* Newbury Park, CA: Sage.

Box, G. E. P., & Jenkins, G. M. (1976). *Time series analysis: Forecasting and control* (rev. ed.). San Francisco: Holden-Day.

Carbonari, J. P., Wirtz, P., Muenz, L., & Stout, R. L. (1994). Alternative analytical methods for detecting matching effects in treatment outcomes. *Journal of Studies on Alcohol, suppl. 12,* 83–90.

Cisler, R., Holder, H. D., Longabaugh, R., Stout, R. L., & Zweben, A. (1998). Actual and estimated replication costs for alcohol treatment modalities: Case study from Project MATCH. *Journal of Studies on Alcohol, 59,* 503–512.

Commentaries. (1999). Comments on Project MATCH: Matching alcohol treatments to patient heterogeneity. *Addiction, 94,* 31–69.

Drummond, D. C. (1999). Treatment research in the wake of Project MATCH. *Addiction, 94,* 39–42.

Finney, J. W., & Monahan, S. C. (1996). The cost effectiveness of treatment for alcoholism: A second approximation. *Journal of Studies on Alcohol, 57,* 229–243.

Folland, S., Goodman, A., & Stano, M. (1993). *The economics of health and health care.* New York: Macmillan.

Godfrey, C. (1999). The "value" of Project MATCH for service provision. *Addiction, 94,* 54–55.

Gold, M. R., Siegel, J. E., Russell, L. B., & Weinstein, M. C. (1996). *Cost-effectiveness in health and medicine.* New York: Oxford University Press.

Holder, H. D. (1998). The cost offsets of alcoholism treatment. In M. Galanter (Ed.), *Recent developments in alcoholism.* Vol. 14: *The consequences of alcoholism* (pp. 361–374). New York: Plenum.

Holder, H. D., & Blose, J. O. (1992). The reduction of health care costs associated with alcoholism treatment: A 14-year longitudinal study. *Journal of Studies on Alcohol, 53,* 293–302.

Holder, H. D., Lennox, R., & Blose, J. O. (1992). The economic benefits of alcoholism treatment: A summary of twenty years of research. *Journal of Employee Assistance Research, 1,* 63–82.

Holder, H. D., Longabaugh, R., Miller, W. R., & Rubonis, A. V. (1991). The cost effectiveness of treatment for alcoholism: A first approximation. *Journal of Studies on Alcohol, 52,* 517–540.

Jones, K. R., & Vischi, J. R. (1979). Impact of alcohol drug abuse and mental health treatment on medical care utilization: A review of the research literature. *Medical Care, 17,* 1–82.

Miller, W. R., Brown, J. M., Simpson, T. L., Handmaker, N. S., Bien, T. H., Luckie, L. F., Montgomery, H. A., Hester, R. K., & Tonigan, J. S. (1995). What works? A methodological analysis of alcoholism treatment outcome literature. In R. H. Hester & W. R. Miller (Eds.), *Handbook of alcoholism treatment approaches: Effective alternatives* (2nd ed., pp. 12–44). New York: Allyn and Bacon.

Project MATCH Research Group. (1997a). Matching alcoholism treatments to patient heterogeneity: Project MATCH posttreatment drinking outcomes. *Journal of Studies on Alcohol, 58,* 7–29.

Project MATCH Research Group. (1997b). Project MATCH secondary a priori hypotheses. *Addiction, 92,* 1671–1698.

Project MATCH Research Group. (1998a). Matching alcoholism treatments to patient heterogeneity: Project MATCH three-year drinking outcomes. *Alcoholism, Clinical and Experimental Research, 22,* 1300–1311.

Project MATCH Research Group. (1998b). Matching patients with alcohol disorders to treatments: Clinical implications from Project MATCH. *Journal of Mental Health, 7,* 589–602.

Chapter 6

Use of Anticonvulsants in Benzodiazepine Withdrawal

Kenneth P. Pages, M.D.
Richard K. Ries, M.D.

THERAPEUTIC USES OF ANXIOLYTICS AND SEDATIVE/HYPNOTICS

Anxiolytics and sedative/hypnotic agents have broad therapeutic uses, including treatment for anxiety disorders, insomnia, alcohol withdrawal syndromes, muscle relaxation, and seizure control. Although the sedative and hypnotic class includes barbiturates and zolpidem, the focus of this article is on benzodiazepines (BZPs). Barbiturates have a well-established liability for psychoactive dependence and a well-established withdrawal syndrome (Morgan, 1990; Sullivan & Sellers, 1986). Zolpidem, a selective omega 1 BZP receptor agonist, used as a hypnotic, does not have a clearly identified potential for abuse or a withdrawal syndrome that has been shown in controlled studies, but there have been case reports of individual patients experiencing withdrawal upon discontinuation of zolpidem (Cavallaro et al., 1993; Gericke & Ludolph, 1994; Monti et al., 1994; Perrault et al., 1992; Sanchez, Sanchez, & Lopez, 1996; Ware et al., 1997; Watsky, 1996).

The variety of therapeutic indications and the relative safety and efficacy of BZPs has made them among the most prescribed medications (Olfson & Pincus, 1994). Along with widespread use has come the problem of BZP dependence, abuse, and withdrawal (Busto & Sellers, 1991; Greenblatt, Miller, & Shader, 1990; Salzman, 1993; Smith & Landry, 1990). The symptoms arising in the context of BZP withdrawal may result from several sources: (a) return of the original symptoms being treated by the BZPs (recurrence), (b) a worsening or rebound of the original symptoms, or (c) a unique withdrawal syndrome associated with dependence on the BZPs. This paper is limited to a discussion of the withdrawal syndrome and the relative merits of the use of anticonvulsant medications for BZP withdrawal treatment.

WHAT CONSTITUTES BENZODIAZEPINE DEPENDENCE?

There has been considerable debate in the literature about the abuse liability of BZPs (Catalan & Gath, 1985; Cole & Chiarello, 1990; DuPont, 1993; Lader, 1994; Moley, Dawkes, & Berry, 1994; Piper, 1995; Woods, Katz, & Winger, 1992). It is important to differentiate physiological dependence from substance abuse or dependence as defined by the DSM-IV (American Psychiatric Association, 1994). The consensus appears to be that most patients will develop iatrogenic physiological dependence on BZPs at even moderate therapeutic doses with chronic use. BZP use becomes a problem when use becomes abuse or psychoactive substance dependence (i.e., "addiction") and the patient shows loss of control, use despite adverse consequences, and compulsion to use. Patients may escalate the dose and/or engage in dysfunctional behavior associated with procuring the medication. It has been shown that abuse becomes more probable when the patient has a previous history of substance abuse problems. Such patients tend to use BZPs in combination with other drugs either to augment the euphoriant effects (Barnas et al., 1992; Darke, Ross, & Hall, 1995) or to counteract the negative effects (Darke, Ross, & Cohen, 1994) of the primary drug. Both patients with a primary indication for BZPs who are iatrogenically physiologically dependent and polysubstance abusers with both physiological and psychoactive substance dependence may need to be withdrawn from BZPs. In the first case, the therapeutic efficacy of the BZPs may be inadequate and different medication trials may be needed, such as selective serotonin reuptake inhibitors (SRIs) for panic disorder. In the second case, withdrawal serves as the first step in facilitating addiction treatment and recovery.

BENZODIAZEPINE WITHDRAWAL SYNDROME

Symptoms of BZP withdrawal range from mild to severe and include anxiety, agitation, sleep disturbances, tremor, perceptual disturbances, paranoia, and seizures (Burrows et al., 1990). Besides withdrawal, patients discontinuing BZPs can experience recurrence and rebound (Greenblatt et al., 1990). Recurrence is the slow return of the originally targeted psychiatric symptoms for which the patient was receiving BZP treatment. These symptoms may return over weeks or months and should be of no greater intensity than the original symptoms. Rebound is a syndrome occurring more rapidly than recurrence. Patients with rebound will experience symptoms within hours to days of BZP discontinuation. Although the symptoms are qualitatively similar to the original symptoms, they may be transiently more intense. Both rebound insomnia and rebound anxiety have been well described (Kales et al., 1986; Rickels et al., 1988). Rebound tends to be self-limited and of short duration. Withdrawal is differentiated from either recurrence or rebound by the prominence of additional autonomic symptoms (Roy-Bryne & Homer, 1988). Although most therapeutic BZP withdrawal syndromes are uncomfortable but not life threatening, there are cases of more severe withdrawal presenting with seizures or delirium reported (Fialip et al., 1987; Zipursky, Baker, & Zimmer, 1985), usually in polysubstance abusers. Finally, some authors have described a controversial protracted withdrawal syndrome that may cause mild autonomic and subjective distress over several weeks or months (Ashton, 1991).

TREATMENT OF BENZODIAZEPINE WITHDRAWAL WITH ANTICONVULSANTS

Relationship to Alcohol Withdrawal

Some studies have demonstrated the effectiveness of anticonvulsants (both carbamazepine and sodium valproate) in treating acute alcohol withdrawal (Bjorkquist et al., 1976; Lambie et al., 1980; Malcolm et al., 1989; Stuppaeck et al., 1990, 1992; Rosenthal, Perkel, Singh, Onand, & Miner, 1998). This has led to the hypothesis that anticonvulsants could be useful in the treatment of BZP withdrawal. The most common method of BZP withdrawal was, and probably still is, a slow taper of the original agent over weeks to months. The need for better treatment for acute BZP withdrawal became more pressing with the appearance of widely used, high-potency, short half-life BZPs such as alprazolam and triazolam (Fyer et al., 1987; Klein, Uhde, & Post, 1986; Zipursky et al., 1985). Also, addiction treatment units could not wait for weeks or months of slow taper and were searching for a more rapid method of BZP withdrawal for high-dose BZP dependence in polysubstance abusers (Ries et al., 1991; Smith & Landry, 1990).

Mechanism of Action

The exact mechanism of action involved in anticonvulsants facilitating BZP detoxification is unknown. Alcohol and barbiturates act at the BZP-chloride ionophore macromolecular complex to facilitate GABAergic transmission (Allen & Harris, 1986). Because it has been shown that compounds that inhibit GABAergic neurotransmission produce significant anxiety-like states in primates (Ninan et al., 1982) and humans (Dorow et al., 1983), it is thought that this GABA BZP-chloride ionophore macromolecular complex may explain certain kinds of anxiety and withdrawal syndromes. Valproate may mimic the action of BZPs at the level of these receptors and thus ameliorate the withdrawal phenomenon (Roy-Byrne & Homer, 1988; Roy-Byrne, Ward, & Donnelly, 1989). Interestingly, carbamazepine's mechanism of action may be different because it appears to exert its effects at the peripheral calcium channel-linked receptor rather than the chloride channel-linked central receptor (Schweizer et al., 1991).

Carbamazepine

The first report of the successful use of anticonvulsants in BZP withdrawal was in a series of three patients on alprazolam for treatment of panic disorder (Klein et al., 1986). All three patients were on greater than 5 mg/day and were withdrawn because of complications: two developed hypomania and one developed tachyphylaxis, resulting in a decision to withdraw him once he reached 9 mg/day. The dose of carbamazepine used was different for each patient but ranged from 600 to 800 mg/day. Withdrawal treatment lasted 2 weeks in all three patients. These studies are summarized in Table 6.1.

Another case series (Ries et al., 1989) described the open treatment of nine patients hospitalized on a university's psychiatric inpatient unit or in a

TABLE 6.1. Studies of Anticonvulsants for Benzodiazepine Withdrawal

Study	Anticonvulsant	Problem	N	Outcome	Comment
Klein, Uhde, & Post (1986)	CBZ	Therapeutic	3	+	DB
Ries, Roy-Byrne, Ward, et al. (1989)	CBZ	Poly + therapeutic	9	++	CS
Ries, Cullison, Horn, et al. (1989)	CBZ	Poly	85	++	CS
Swantek, Grossberg, Neppe, et al. (1991)	CBZ	Therapeutic	4	+	CS
Schweizer, Rickels, Case, et al. (1991)	CBZ	Therapeutic	40	+	DB
Garcia Borreguero, Bronisch, Apelt, et al. (1991)	CBZ	Therapeutic	18	+	Open
Klein, Colin, Stolk, et al. (1994)	CBZ	Therapeutic	70	+	Open
Apelt & Emrich (1990)	Valproate	Therapeutic	4	+	CS
Roy-Byrne, Ward, & Donnelly (1989)	Valproate	Therapeutic	1	+	CS
McElroy & Keck (1991)	Vaproate	Therapeutic	1	+	CS

Note: CS = case study; Poly = polysubstance abuse; DB = double blind; Open = open trial.

private substance abuse treatment center. Patients were taking high doses of BZPs (e.g., 2,000 mg/day chlordiazepoxide, 8 mg/day clonazepam, 15 mg/day alprazolam), which were tapered and stopped over a few days as carbamazepine was rapidly initiated. Psychiatric diagnoses, dose of BZP, starting dose of carbamazepine, and rate of taper varied among patients, but all patients also qualified for a diagnosis of psychoactive substance dependence. The authors concluded, based on the absence of treatment with supplemental BZPs during the taper, that carbamazepine provided a more rapid and better tolerated discontinuation from BZPs than a taper alone.

The initial positive results found in the use of carbamazepine to treat BZP withdrawal led to the development of a standardized protocol by Ries et al. (1991). Two slightly different protocols were put into use at two substance detoxification and rehabilitation centers. In order for patients to be included in the study, BZPs had to be the primary drug of abuse; in addition, all patients had to qualify for psychoactive substance dependence. Eighty-five patients were included in the study. In one protocol, a 3-day tapering dose of BZPs was given along with a loading dose of 600 mg/day of carbamazepine. In the other protocol, no regularly scheduled BZPs were given after admission and initiation of the loading dose of carbamazepine. Both of these protocols were rated as better or much better by staff than the previous methods of detoxification (slow taper of BZPs or the use of phenobarbital). The rate of side effects was stated to be the same for taper plus carbamazepine as carbamazepine alone, though specific side effects were not reported.

Carbamazepine has also been used in the treatment of geriatric patients in whom BZP withdrawal is anticipated to be difficult (Swantek et al., 1991). Four elderly patients (average age 72.5 years) hospitalized on a university psychiatric service were withdrawn from therapeutic dependence on alprazolam with carbamazepine. All four were started on 400 mg/day, with two of the patients' dosages going up to 500 mg/day over the course of the taper that occurred over a period of 2–6 days. These patients had a lower average dose of alprazolam, with no patient on more than 2.5 mg/day, but all the patients had been treated with alprazolam for at least 7 months. Of note, these four patients had previously been unable to successfully taper alprazolam. The authors did not identify these patients as psychoactive substance dependent. All four patients were successfully tapered and experienced only mild withdrawal symptoms. The authors concluded that while this taper method was worthy of further investigation and may be a useful tool in the geriatric population, such treatment should only occur on an inpatient unit.

There has been only one double-blind, placebo-controlled trial comparing gradual taper of BZP with and without carbamazepine. Schweizer et al. (1991) studied 40 patients with a history of difficulty discontinuing long-term therapeutic BZPs. They were randomly assigned to treatment with carbamazepine (200 to 800 mg/day) or placebo. A taper of 25% per week was then attempted. There were significant differences in ability of patients to stay off BZPs (in favor of the carbamazepine group) between groups at 5 weeks, but only trend-level differences at 12 weeks. Patient-reported severity of withdrawal symptoms was also different at the trend level favoring patients on carbamazepine. Overall, this study's findings were not as robust as some of the initial open trials would have suggested. Possible explanations include small sample size, high pretreatment dropout rate of patients on higher doses of BZP, relatively low dose of starting carbamazepine, extended pretreatment with carbamazepine, and extended BZP taper.

An open trial using similar methods as the above study gradually tapered nine therapeutic BZP patients while another group of nine patients received additional carbamazepine (Garcia Borreguero et al., 1991). This study was able to show a statistically significant difference between groups favoring the carbamazepine group when comparing severity of withdrawal symptoms. Specifically, measures of withdrawal using the Benzodiazepine Withdrawal Symptoms Questionnaire (BWSQ-2) and a brief anxiety rating scale of the Comprehensive Psychopathological Rating Scale were less severe in the carbamazepine-treated group.

Finally, Klein et al. (1994) examined the possibility that patients with panic disorder are especially vulnerable to alprazolam withdrawal symptoms. Patients with generalized anxiety disorder and panic disorder entered a controlled discontinuation phase after 2 months of open treatment with alprazolam. There were 36 patients in the panic disorder group and 35 patients in the generalized anxiety group. Carbamazepine or placebo was added in a randomized, double-blind fashion, followed by a 25% dose reduction every 3rd day after 1 week. Panic disorder patients encountered more withdrawal problems than patients with generalized anxiety disorder and seemed to benefit more from the addition of carbamazepine.

Valproate

Less has been written about the use of sodium valproate in the treatment of BZP withdrawal. This is puzzling given its promise in the treatment of panic disorder patients (Keck, McElroy, & Friedman, 1992), a group particularly vulnerable to both the withdrawal effects of BZPs (Klein et al., 1994) and symptom recurrence and rebound. A small series (Apelt & Emrich, 1990) and two case reports suggest a positive role for valproate in the treatment of BZP withdrawal syndrome.

Apelt and Emrich (1990) reported the treatment of four patients solely dependent on BZPs treated with valproate for protracted withdrawal symptoms. The four patients had different psychiatric disorders, and one had a history of alcohol abuse. These were all patients on high, chronic doses of BZPs, up to 25 mg of lorazepam for anywhere from 1 to 18 years. All four patients had successful attenuation of their withdrawal.

Roy-Byrne et al. (1989) reported a case of a 44-year-old man who had been on alprazolam (2–5 mg/day) for over 3 years. Two initial attempts to taper the patient's alprazolam had been unsuccessful. Both attempts were with a tapering method, one with alprazolam and the other with clonazepam. The patient reported increased depression, tremulousness, and mood swings with each attempted taper. The third attempt at discontinuation of alprazolam involved the use of valproate. This case was unusual because the patient had a primary diagnosis of bipolar disorder and had been on valproate for 10 months before tapering of alprazolam. The patient was successfully tapered ultimately, and the authors commented that 6 months later the patient remained BZP-free and was completely medication-free for 4 months.

McElroy, Keck, and Lawrence (1991) treated a 23-year-old male with severe treatment-resistant panic disorder complicated by apparent clonazepam-induced interdose rebound and/or withdrawal symptoms. This patient had initially been treated with diazepam (90 mg/day). An attempted taper of the diazepam resulted in an abrupt increase in daily panic and generalized anxiety (55 mg/day), and the patient was hospitalized for evaluation and BZP detoxification. Clonazepam was substituted over a 3-day period with a final dose of 12 mg/day given over four doses. The patient continued to complain of a generalized anxiety that increased during the hour before his dose of clonazepam. Attempts at reduction of clonazepam brought a marked worsening of symptoms. Valproate was added with titration to 2,000 mg/day (serum level 89 g/ml). The patient's anxiety lifted, and taper of clonazepam was again attempted at a rate of 1 mg every 3 days. When his dose of clonazepam reached 1 mg/day, he complained of recurrent panic attacks, and his valproate was increased to a total daily dose of 2,250 mg. Clonazepam was then discontinued without incident.

SUMMARY

The evidence is good that anticonvulsants, particularly carbamazepine, help alleviate the symptoms of BZP withdrawal. To date, most of these studies have been clinical rather than randomized, and there have been a number of case reports. It is puzzling that more research has not been supported given that anticonvulsants are not abused and appear to allow rapid discontinuation of BZPs. This point is especially applicable in the case of outpatient detoxification and suggests the development of protocols to evaluate use of anticonvulsants compared to the use of a slow BZP taper.

Although most published reports have involved carbamazepine, carbamazepine also has more side effects than valproate and other new anticonvulsants, specifically gabapentin. Also, because valproate may potentially treat both BZP dependence and symptom recurrence/rebound (e.g., panic attacks, mania), more research is needed to better evaluate valproate in both therapeutic and substance-abusing BZP-dependent populations.

Finally, there may be an important difference between patients dependent on BZPs as part of their polydrug addiction and those dependent on BZPs for therapeutic purposes, such as panic disorder. It appears that patients with psychoactive substance dependence tolerate a rapid anticonvulsant dose escalation and BZP taper (e.g., 1–3 days; Allen & Harris, 1986; Ries et al., 1991) much better than patients who are iatrogenically dependent. Further, because therapeutically dependent patients will need both treatment for BZP withdrawal and replacement treatment for their primary anxiety disorder, the use of agents such as valproate, which may have beneficial effects for both, need further study. Given the pressure of managed care for briefer inpatient stays and the use of outpatient detoxification, it is surprising that there has been so little rigorous research in what appears to be a promising area.

REFERENCES

Allen, A. M., & Harris, R. A. (1986). Involvement of neuronal chloride channels in ethanol intoxication, tolerance and dependence. In M. Galanter (Ed.), *Recent developments in alcoholism* (Vol. 5, pp 313–325). New York: Plenum.

American Psychiatric Association. (1994). *Diagnostic and statistical manual of mental disorders* (4th ed.). Washington, DC: Author.

Apelt, S., & Emrich, H. M. (1990). Sodium valproate in benzodiazepine withdrawal [letter]. *American Journal of Psychiatry, 147,* 950–951.

Ashton, H. (1991). Protracted withdrawal syndromes from benzodiazepines. *Journal of Substance Abuse Treatment, 8,* 19–28.

Barnas, C., Rossmann, M., Roessier, H., et al. (1992). Benzodiazepines and other psychotropic drugs abused by patients in a methadone maintenance program: Familiarity and preference. *Journal of Clinical Psychopharmacology, 12,* 397–402.

Bjorkqvist, S. E., Isohanni, M., Makeja, R., et al. (1976). Ambulant treatment of alcohol withdrawal symptoms with carbamazepine: A formal multicenter double-blind comparison with placebo. *Acta Psychiatrica Scandinavica, 53,* 333–342.

Burrows, G. D., Norman, T. R., Judd, F. K., et al. (1990). Short-acting versus long-acting benzodiazepines: Discontinuation effects in panic disorders. *Journal of Psychiatric Research, 24*(suppl. 2), 65–72.

Busto, U. E., & Sellers, E. M. (1991). Anxiolytics and sedative/hypnotics dependence. *British Journal of Addiction, 86,* 1647–1652.

Catalan, J., & Gath, C. H. (1985). Benzodiazepines in general practice: Time for a decision. *BMJ, 290,* 406–411.

Cavallaro, R., Regazetti, M. G., Covelli, G., et al. (1993). Tolerance and withdrawal with zolpidem. *Lancet, 342,* 374–375.

Cole, J. O., & Chiarello, R. J. (1990). The benzodiazepines as drugs of abuse. *Journal of Psychiatric Research, 24*(suppl. 2), 135–144.

Darke, S. G., Ross, J., & Cohen, J. (1994). The use of benzodiazepines among regular amphetamine users. *Addiction, 89,* 1683–1690.

Darke, S. G., Ross, J. E., & Hall, W. D. (1995). Benzodiazepine use among injecting heroin users. *Medical Journal of Australia, 162,* 645–647.

Dorow, R., Horowski, R., Pashelke, G., et al. (1983). Severe anxiety induced by FG 7142, a beta-carboline ligand for benzodiazepine receptors. *Lancet, 2,* 98–99.

DuPont, R. L. (1993). Benzodiazepines, addiction, and public policy. *New Jersey Medicine, 90,* 823–826.

Fialip, J., Aumaitre, O., Eschalier, A., et al. (1987). Benzodiazepine withdrawal seizures: Analysis of 48 case reports. *Clinical Neuropharmacology, 10,* 538–544.

Fyer, A. J., Liebowitz, M. R., Gorman, J. M., et al. (1987). Discontinuation of alprazolam treatment in panic patients. *American Journal of Psychiatry, 144,* 303–308.

Garcia Borreguero, D., Bronisch, T., Apelt, S., et al. (1991). Treatment of benzodiazepine withdrawal symptoms with carbamazepine. *European Archives of Psychiatry and Clinical Neuroscience, 241,* 145–150.

Gericke, C. A., & Ludolph, A. C. (1994). Chronic abuse of zolpidem. *Journal of the American Medical Association, 272,* 1721–1722.

Greenblatt, D. J., Miller, L. G., & Shader, R. I. (1990). Benzodiazepine discontinuation syndromes. *Journal of Psychiatric Research, 24*(Suppl. 2), 73–79.

Kales, A., Bixler, E. O., Vela-Bueno, A., et al. (1986). Comparison of short and long half-life benzodiazepine hypnotics: triazolam and quazepam. *Clinical Pharmacology and Therapeutics, 40,* 378–386.

Keck, P. E. J., McElroy, S. L., & Friedman, L. M. (1992). Valproate and carbamazepine in the treatment of panic and posttraumatic stress disorders, withdrawal states, and behavioral dyscontrol syndromes. *Journal of Clinical Psychopharmacology, 12*(suppl. 1), 36S–41S.

Klein, E., Colin, V., Stolk, J., et al. (1994). Alprazolam withdrawal in patients with panic disorder and generalized anxiety disorder: Vulnerability and effect of carbamazepine. *American Journal of Psychiatry, 151,* 1760–1766.

Klein, E., Uhde, T. W., & Post, R. M. (1986). Preliminary evidence for the utility of carbamazepine in alprazolam withdrawal. *American Journal of Psychiatry, 143,* 235–236.

Lader, M. (1994). Anxiolytic drugs: Dependence, addiction and abuse. *European Neuropsychopharmacology, 4,* 85–91.

Lambie, D. G., Johnson, M. E., Vijayasenan, E. A., et al. (1980). Sodium valproate in the treatment of the alcohol withdrawal syndrome. *Australian and New Zealand Journal of Psychiatry, 14,* 213–215.

Malcolm, R., Ballenger, J. C., Sturgis, E. T., et al. (1989). Double-blind controlled trial comparing carbamazepine to oxazepam treatment of alcohol withdrawal. *American Journal of Psychiatry, 146,* 617–621.

McElroy, S. L., Keck, P. E. J., & Lawrence, J. M. (1991). Treatment of panic disorder and benzodiazepine withdrawal with valproate [letter]. *Journal of Neuropsychiatry and Clinical Neuroscience, 3,* 232–233.

Moley, F. M., Dawkes, M., & Berry, J. P. (1994). Misuse of benzodiazepines: Avoid benzodiazepines whenever possible [letter; comment]. *BMJ, 308,* 1709–1710.

Monti, J. M., Attali, P., Monti, D., et al. (1994). Zolpidem and rebound insomnia—a double-blind, controlled polysomnographic study in chronic insomniac patients. *Pharmacopsychiatry, 27,* 166–175.

Morgan, W. W. (1990). Abuse liability of barbiturates and other sedative-hypnotics. *Advances in Alcohol and Substance Abuse, 9,* 67–82.

Ninan, P. T., Insel, T. M., Cohen, R. W., et al. (1982). Benzodiazepine receptor-mediated experimental anxiety in primates. *Science, 218,* 1332–1334.

Olfson, M., & Pincus, H. A. (1994). Use of benzodiazepines in the community. *Archives of Internal Medicine, 154,* 1235–1240.

Perrault, G., Morel, E., Sanger, D. J., et al. (1992). Lack of tolerance and physical dependence upon repeated treatment with the novel hypnotic zolpidem. *Journal of Pharmacology and Experimental Therapeutics, 263,* 298–303.

Piper, A. (1995). Addiction to benzodiazepines—how common? [see comments]. *Archives of Family Medicine, 4,* 964–970.

Rickels, K., Fox, I. L., Greenblatt, D. J., et al. (1988). Clorazepate and lorazepam: Clinical improvement and rebound anxiety. *American Journal of Psychiatry, 145,* 312–317.

Ries, R. K., Roy-Byrne, P. P., Ward, N. G., et al. (1989). Carbamazepine treatment for benzodiazepine withdrawal. *American Journal of Psychiatry, 146,* 536–537.

Ries, R., Cullison, S., Horn, R., et al. (1991). Benzodiazepine withdrawal: Clinicians' ratings of carbamazepine treatment versus traditional taper methods. *Journal of Psychoactive Drugs, 23,* 73–76.

Rosenthal, R. N., Perkel, C., Singh, P., Anand, O., & Miner, C. R. (1998). A pilot open randomized trial of valproate and phenobarbital in the treatment of acute alcohol withdrawal. *The American Journal on Addictions, 7,* 189–197.

Roy-Byrne, P. P., & Homer, D. (1988). Benzodiazepine withdrawal: an overview and implications for the treatment of anxiety. *American Journal of Medicine, 84,* 1041–1052.

Roy-Byrne, P. P., Ward, N. G., & Donnelly, P. J. (1989). Valproate in anxiety and withdrawal syndromes. *Journal of Clinical Psychiatry, 50,* 44–48.

Salzman, C. (1993). Benzodiazepine treatment of panic and agoraphobic symptoms: Use, dependence, toxicity, abuse. *Journal of Psychiatric Research, 27*(suppl. 1), 97–110.

Sanchez, L. G., Sanchez, J. M., & Lopez, M.-J. (1996). Dependence and tolerance with zolpidem. *American Journal of Health-System Pharmacy, 53,* 2638.

Schweizer, E., Rickels, K., Case, W. G., et al. (1991). Carbamazepine treatment in patients discontinuing long-term benzodiazepine therapy: Effects on withdrawal severity and outcome. *Archives of General Psychiatry, 48,* 448–452.

Smith, D. E., & Landry, M. J. (1990). Benzodiazepine dependency discontinuation: Focus on the chemical dependency detoxification setting and benzodiazepine-polydrug abuse. *Journal of Psychiatric Research, 24*(suppl. 2), 145–156.

Stuppaeck, C. H., Barnas, C., Hackenberg, K., et al. (1990). Carbamazepine monotherapy in the treatment of alcohol withdrawal. *International Clinical Psychopharmacology, 5,* 273–278.

Stuppaeck, C. H., Pycha, R., C. M., et al. (1992). Carbamazepine versus oxazepam in the treatment of alcohol withdrawal: A double-blind study. *Alcohol and Alcoholism, 27,* 153–158.

Sullivan, J. T., & Sellers, E. M. (1986). Treatment of the barbiturate abstinence syndrome. *Medical Journal of Australia, 145,* 456–458.

Swantek, S. S., Grossberg, G. T., Neppe, V. M., et al. (1991). The use of carbamazepine to treat benzodiazepine withdrawal in a geriatric population. *Journal of Geriatric Psychiatry and Neurology, 4,* 106–109.

Ware, J. C., Walsh, J. K., Scharf, M. B., et al. (1997). Minimal rebound insomnia after treatment with 10-mg zolpidem. *Clinical Neuropharmacology, 20,* 116–125.

Watsky, E. (1996). Management of zolpidem withdrawal. *Journal of Clinical Psychopharmacology, 16,* 459.

Woods, J. H., Katz, J. I., & Winger, G. (1992). Benzodiazepines: Use, abuse, and consequences. *Pharmacological Reviews, 44,* 151–347.

Zipursky, R. B., Baker, R. W., & Zimmer, B. (1985). Alprazolam withdrawal delirium unresponsive to diazepam: Case report. *Journal of Clinical Psychiatry, 46,* 344–345.

Chapter 7

Pharmacologic Treatment of Heroin-Dependent Patients

Patrick G. O'Connor, M.D., M.P. H.
David A. Fiellin, M.D.

Illicit drug use is responsible for more than 25,000 deaths and $100 billion in total economic costs annually in the United States (Harwood, Fountain, & Livermore, 1998). Recently, heroin has emerged as the major contributor to these societal problems and costs. Persons suffering from heroin abuse and dependence are an important patient population for general internists. Although patients may present with medical problems that relate directly to heroin or its route of administration (for example, injection), physicians are often unaware of the underlying drug abuse problems (Schorling & Buchsbaum, 1997) and thus may miss the opportunity to offer drug treatment services. Over the past decade, research on heroin dependence has demonstrated that treatment is effective, and new pharmacologically based treatments show promise for the expansion of treatment options (Kosten & McCance, 1996). Most recently, research has suggested that internists may have a direct role in the provision of drug treatment services for heroin-dependent persons in their offices (O'Connor et al., 1998). In this chapter, we review the treatment of heroin dependence and emphasize recent developments in pharmacologically based treatment approaches.

Dr. Feillin is supported by the National Institute on Drug Abuse Physician Scientist Award (K12 DA00167).

METHODS

All relevant English-language articles identified through the MEDLINE database from 1968 through January 2000 were systematically searched by using the following key words: *heroin, heroin dependence, narcotics, opioids, substance-related disorders, substance withdrawal syndrome,* and *narcotic antagonists.* Selected references from these articles and appropriate textbooks were also reviewed.

DEFINITIONS AND EPIDEMIOLOGY

The most commonly used terms to describe the clinical phenomena of illicit drug use (as well as use of nonillicit substances) are *substance abuse* and *substance dependence* (Table 7.1; American Psychiatric Association, 1994). Thus,

TABLE 7.1. *Diagnostic and Statistical Manual of Mental Disorders-IV* Criteria for Substance Abuse and Dependence[a]

Substance abuse: A maladaptive pattern of substance use leading to clinical impairment or distress in those who never met criteria for dependence in the past, manifested within a 12-month period by one or more of the following characteristics:
>   Recurrent use resulting in a failure to fulfill role obligations at work, school, or home
>   Recurrent use in physically hazardous situations, such as driving or operating machines
>   Recurrent substance-related legal problems (for example, arrests)
>   Continued use despite social or interpersonal problems (for example, physical fights, marital problems)

Substance dependence: A maladaptive pattern of substance use leading to clinical impairment or distress, manifested within a 12-month period by three or more of the following characteristics:
>   Tolerance, defined by increased amounts used to achieve intoxication or other desired effect or diminished effects with continued use of the same amount of the substance
>   Withdrawal, manifested by the characteristic withdrawal syndrome, or use of the substance to relieve or avoid withdrawal symptoms
>   Substance taken in larger amounts or over a longer period than intended
>   Persistent desire or unsuccessful attempts to cut down or control substance use
>   Great deal of time spent obtaining the substance, using the substance, or recovering from the effects of substance use
>   Important social, occupational, recreational activities given up or reduced
>   Substance use despite knowledge of associated physical or psychological problems

[a]Adapted from APA (1994).

these criteria are used when diagnosing opioid abuse and opioid dependence. Heroin, a pure opioid agonist derived from morphine, was initially manufactured in the 1800s for use as an antitussive. Currently, illicit heroin is sold as a white or brownish powder in "bags" or "bundles" (10 bags) and is commonly mixed ("cut") with adulterants, such as sugar or quinine. The availability of increasingly pure heroin has been responsible for an increased incidence of heroin overdose in some locations (Hamid et al., 1997). Increased purity and the risk for HIV infection have resulted in a shift from heroin injection to smoking (Schottenfeld, O'Malley, Abdul-Salaam, & O'Connor, 1993). According to the 1997 National Household Survey on Drug Abuse, approximately 2.5 million Americans have used heroin, and the number of persons reporting heroin use over the past month increased fivefold between 1993 and 1997. In addition, data from the 1996 Drug Abuse Warning Network (DAWN) survey documented a 108% increase in heroin-related emergency department episodes between 1990 and 1996.

COMMON CLINICAL PROBLEMS IN HEROIN-DEPENDENT PATIENTS

Heroin-dependent patients are at risk for a wide variety of medical, psychiatric, and behavioral health problems. Thus, patients should be routinely screened in clinical practice for heroin abuse and dependence, as well as other substance use disorders (Schorling & Buchsbaum, 1997). Although well-accepted screening instruments (for example, the CAGE questionnaire) have been developed and tested for identifying patients with alcohol use disorders, no parallel instruments have been as rigorously tested for the identification of heroin abuse and dependence (U.S. Preventive Services Task Force, 1996). However, modifications of existing instruments (for example, the CAGE-D) have been developed and are under evaluation (Schorling & Buchsbaum). In the meantime, routine inquiry about past and current use of heroin and other drugs should be performed in all patients. Additional questions on symptoms related to heroin use (such as overdose and withdrawal), routes of administration, and complications associated with heroin use should be asked if indicated.

The medical problems that may result from heroin use are numerous and have been discussed in detail elsewhere (Cherubin & Sapira, 1993; O'Connor, Selwyn, & Schottenfeld, 1994; Sporer, 1999; Stein, 1990). Psychiatric comorbidity is also highly prevalent among persons who use drugs (Ziedonis & Brady, 1997). In a study of 716 treatment-seeking opioid abusers, 47% were found to have psychiatric comorbid conditions (including personality disorders, depression, and anxiety disorders), and psychiatric problems were associated with more severe substance abuse problems; Brooner, King, Kidorf, Schmidt, & Bigelow, 1997; Darke & Ross, 1997). Heroin users are also at high risk for abusing other substances, including benzodiazepines, alcohol, and cocaine

(Brooner et al., 1997; Chutuape, Brooner, & Stitzer, 1997). The problem of dependence on multiple substances can be particularly vexing for patients, physicians, and drug treatment programs, given the complexity of multiple drug effects (for example, different patterns of dependence and withdrawal) seen in these patients. In addition, unlike with heroin, no pharmacologic agent has been demonstrated to effectively treat cocaine dependence (Warner, Kosten, & O'Connor, 1997). Thus, because many opioid-abusing patients concurrently use other drugs with heroin, such as cocaine and alcohol, physicians need to keep in mind that heroin detoxification and methadone maintenance do not necessarily effectively treat withdrawal or reduce the use of other drugs in these patients.

Other behavior-related problems, such as family dysfunction, unemployment, and legal problems, are highly prevalent among heroin-dependent patients (Wyshak & Modest, 1996). In addition, accidents and injuries, criminal behavior, and domestic violence are associated with illicit drug use (Regidor, Barrio, de la Fuente, & Rodriguez, 1996; Liebschutz, Mulrey, & Samet, 1997; Brewer, Fleming, Haggerty, & Catalano, 1998).

Because of the wide variety of health problems experienced by heroin-dependent patients, internists are in a unique position to provide enhanced screening and preventive health services to these patients. This includes screening for medical conditions, such as HIV disease and hepatitis; provision of appropriate vaccinations; screening for psychiatric problems, including depression; and assessment for behavior-related problems, such as high-risk sexual activity or physical abuse (Table 7.2). Patients identified as having psychiatric, behavioral, or physical abuse problems should be referred for appropriate services as indicated. Similarly, social complications should be addressed by referral to social work, family counseling, or other social service agencies if needed.

TREATMENT APPROACHES FOR PATIENTS WITH HEROIN DEPENDENCE

Heroin-dependent patients require a thoughtful management approach if they are to be successfully engaged in substance abuse treatment. Once such patients are identified, it is critical for the physican to assess patients' readiness to change their drug-using behaviors (Prochaska, DiClemente, Velicer, & Rossi, 1992). Prochaska and DiClemente's six-stage model describing the stages of patients' readiness to change their behaviors has been widely accepted as useful for guiding physicians' initial treatment approach (Prochaska et al., 1992; Samet, Rollinick, & Barnes, 1996). In the "precontemplation" stage, patients are not thinking of their substance use as problematic and are thus unlikely to see a need for treatment. Physicians must help patients overcome denial and

TABLE 7.2. Routine Screening and Prevention Activities for Clinicians
Caring for Drug Users[a]

Complication	Screening or Prevention Activity
Medical	
Bacterial infection	Pneumococcal vaccine
Viral infection	HIV counseling and testing
	HIV staging and therapy (if appropriate)
	Screening for hepatitis A, B, and C
	Vaccination against hepatitis A and B
	Vaccination against influenza
Sexually transmitted diseases	Screening for syphillis, gonorrhea, and chlamydia
Tuberculosis	Screening for infection and active disease
Malignant conditions	Screening for cervical cancer
	Screening for other cancer (as indicated)
Psychiatric	
Depression	Assessment for symptoms
Anxiety and other problems	Assessment for symptoms
Other substance abuse	CAGE questionnaire (alcohol problems)
	Assessment for use of other illicit drugs (for example, cocaine)
	Assessment for abuse of prescription drugs
Behavioral	
Accidents and injuries	Assessment for symptoms, signs
Physical or sexual abuse	Assessment for symptoms, signs
Social	
Unemployment, homelessness	Assessment of living situation
Lack of entitlements	Assessment of resources to support medical care

[a]CAGE = cut down, annoyed, guilty, eye-opener.

move them into the "precontemplation," "contemplation," and "determination" stages rather than referring them to treatment that they believe they do not need (Samet et al., 1996). After a patient has entered the "action" phase, physician support for behavior change and treatment is crucial. Of interest is that one study of primary care patients who screened positive for alcohol abuse and dependence determined that 63% of patients were in the "action" phase (Samet & O'Connor, 1998). This suggests that supporting relapse prevention is a very important role for physicians (Friedmann, Saitz, & Samet, 1998).

Once patients indicate an interest in treatment, their appropriateness for opioid detoxification or opioid agonist maintenance should be determined. We discuss these two aspects of treatment in detail and emphasize pharmacologic approaches to detoxification and maintenance.

HEROIN WITHDRAWAL: DIAGNOSIS AND MANAGEMENT

The Opioid Withdrawal Syndrome

The opioid withdrawal syndrome consists of signs and symptoms that result in part from neurophysiologic rebound in the organ systems affected by opioids. These systems (and signs and symptoms) include the cardiovascular system (tachycardia, hypertension), central nervous system (pupillary dilatation, restlessness, irritability, insomnia, craving), gastrointestinal system (nausea, vomiting, diarrhea), skin (piloerection), and mucous membranes (rhinorrhea, lacrimation). Although no widely accepted assessment instrument is available for managing opioid withdrawal, brief, easy-to-use assessment tools that may be useful in clinical practice have been developed (Gossop, 1990). Unlike patients undergoing alcohol withdrawal, patients experiencing opioid withdrawal do not typically have such severe complications as seizures, arrhythmias, or delirium tremens. In opioid withdrawal, both subjective (for example, craving) and objective (for example, vomiting) phenomena, especially intense craving, frequently lead to relapse. Thus, the effective management of opioid withdrawal is a critical first step in treating patients. Subsequent referral of detoxified patients to ongoing drug treatment services is also essential for proper and effective management.

The time of onset, peak symptoms, and duration of opioid withdrawal vary, depending on the specific opioid drug being used. For example, symptoms of heroin withdrawal usually begin 4 to 6 hours after last use, peak within approximately 24 to 48 hours, and may last for 7 to 14 days. In contrast, symptoms of withdrawal from methadone, a longer-acting opioid, generally begin 24 to 36 hours after last use and can last for several days to a few weeks. The management of opioid withdrawal combines general supportive measures and pharmacologic treatments. Supportive measures include a safe environment, adequate nutrition, and careful monitoring. Pharmacologic therapies, including opioids and nonopioids, can be provided to alleviate withdrawal symptoms.

Detoxification Using Opioid Agonists

Opioid-based detoxification is based on the principle of cross-tolerance, in which one opioid is replaced with another that is slowly tapered. Methadone is used because it has a long half-life and can be administered once daily. Withdrawal from heroin is usually managed with initial dosages of methadone in the range of 15 to 30 mg per day (Fultz & Senay, 1975; Tennant, Russell, Casas, & Bleich, 1975). Although this dosage is generally adequate to control symptoms in many heroin users over a 24-hour period, additional methadone can be given as required on the basis of clinical findings. In acute medical settings, this dosage should be maintained through the second or third day and then slowly tapered by approximately 10% to 15% per day. Longer term opioid detoxification using methadone is often available through drug treatment programs. Although a licensed physician can perform methadone detoxification in an inpatient medical setting, outpatient detoxification requires a specially licensed drug treatment program.

More recently, buprenorphine, a partial opioid agonist, has been studied as a treatment for opioid withdrawal. One study randomly assigned 45 heroin-dependent patients to buprenorphine (2 mg) or methadone (30 mg) for 3 weeks, followed by tapering over a 4-week period, and found both approaches to be equivalent (Bickel et al., 1988). Another study that compared a gradual (36 days) to a more rapid (12 days) buprenorphine taper (initially 8 mg) found the gradual approach to be superior (Amass, Bickel, Higgins, & Hughes, 1994). A study that compared a 3-day course of buprenorphine (3 mg) to a 5-day course of clonidine reported that these approaches were equivalent (Cheskin, Fudala, & Johnson, 1994), although another study found that a longer course of buprenorphine (10 days) was superior to clonidine (Nigam, Ray, & Tripathi, 1993).

Detoxification Using Nonopioid Medications

Nonopioid methods of opioid detoxification have focused primarily on clonidine, an α_2-agonist, which diminishes norepinephrine activity during opioid withdrawal (Gossop, 1988). Early studies demonstrated that clonidine diminished withdrawal symptoms in patients who were withdrawn from methadone (Charney, Sternberg, Kleber, Heninger, & Redmond, 1981; Kleber et al., 1985). Clonidine seems to be most effective in suppressing autonomic signs and symptoms of opioid withdrawal but is less effective for subjective withdrawal symptoms (Rosen et al., 1996). Initial daily doses of up to 1.2 mg in divided doses are commonly suggested. For example, a regimen of 0.1 to 0.2 mg every 4 hours has been used in two clinical trials for heroin withdrawal, with careful monitoring of blood pressure (O'Connor et al., 1995, 1997). Because it may be less effective in managing subjective withdrawal symptoms, adjuvant therapy (nonsteroidal anti-inflammatory drugs for myalgia, benzodiazepines for insomnia, and antiemetics) may be needed (O'Connor et al., 1995, 1997).

Although methadone is most commonly used for opioid withdrawal in pregnancy, data from one study suggest that clonidine may be appropriate for some pregnant women with mild withdrawal (Dashe, Jackson, Olscher, Zane, & Wendel, 1998). In addition, in a randomized trial that included 55 patients who received clonidine in a primary care setting, 65% of patients underwent successful detoxification (O'Connor et al., 1997). In another study that examined predictors of successful clonidine detoxification, patients who completed detoxification were more likely to be heroin smokers (rather than intravenous users) and to have abstained from opioids for a longer time before presenting for treatment (McCann et al., 1997).

Lofexidine, a centrally acting α_2-adrenergic agonist, has also been evaluated as a treatment for opioid withdrawal, although it has not yet been approved by the U.S. Food and Drug Administration (FDA) for this purpose. In a randomized trial that compared lofexidine to methadone in 86 opioid addicts, lofexidine-treated patients had more severe withdrawal symptoms from Days 3 to 7 and again on Day 10 but had similar symptoms thereafter. Rates of treatment completion did not significantly differ (Bearn, Gossop, & Strang, 1996). In two randomized, double-blind trials that compared lofexidine with clonidine in patients dependent on methadone (Kahn, Mumford, Rogers, & Beckford, 1997) and heroin (Lin, Strang, Su, Tsai, & Hu, 1997), both agents effectively reduced withdrawal symptoms. Patients treated with lofexidine experienced fewer side effects, especially hypotension. Finally, one study suggested that a 5-day lofexidine regimen decreased symptoms of opioid withdrawal more rapidly than a 10-day regimen (Bearn, Gossop, & Strang, 1998).

Rapid and Ultrarapid Opioid Detoxification

Because most opioid and nonopioid approaches to detoxification require a prolonged time frame of a week or more, "rapid" and "ultrarapid" opioid detoxification protocols have been developed (O'Connor & Kosten, 1998). These protocols use an opioid antagonist (for example, naloxone or naltrexone) to cause an accelerated withdrawal response, with the goal of completing detoxification in time periods from 8 days to as little as a few hours. In addition to an opioid antagonist, both approaches use pharmacotherapies (for example, clonidine, sedation, and general anesthesia) to minimize the acute withdrawal symptoms experienced when opioid antagonists are administered. Because detoxification is completed more quickly, these approaches may have the advantage of minimizing the risk for relapse and allowing patients to enter postdetoxification treatments, such as naltrexone maintenance, more rapidly.

Rapid Opioid Detoxification

Rapid opioid detoxification was first described by Resnick, Kestenbaum, Washton, and Poole (1977) in a cohort of 29 methadone-dependent patients who were given naloxone and began naltrexone maintenance within 48 hours in an inpatient setting. Rapid detoxification with naltrexone was first studied by Charney, Heninger, and Kleber (1986) in 40 methadone-maintained patients who were also treated as inpatients. Kleber, Topazian, Gaspari, Riordan, and Kosten (1987) performed the first study of rapid detoxification in heroin-dependent patients in an outpatient substance abuse treatment unit. Most of the 14 participants in this study (86%) successfully began naltrexone maintenance (Kleber et al., 1987).

O'Connor and colleagues examined rapid detoxification in a "primary care" setting in two studies that compared the procedure with clonidine

(O'Connor et al., 1995, 1997). In the first study, in which patients selected their treatment, 94% (60 of 64 patients) in the rapid detoxification group successfully completed detoxification compared with 42% (24 of 57 patients) in the clonidine group (O'Connor et al., 1995). In a subsequent randomized clinical trial of 162 patients that compared two methods of rapid detoxification with clonidine, more patients (81%) successfully completed detoxification in the two rapid detoxification groups than in the clonidine group (65%), although the difference did not achieve statistical significance (O'Connor et al., 1997). In addition, this study demonstrated that patients who were treated with a rapid detoxification protocol that used buprenorphine experienced less severe withdrawal than did patients in the other two groups (O'Connor et al., 1997).

Ultrarapid Opioid Detoxification

Ultrarapid detoxification was first described in a study of 12 opioid-dependent patients who were given naloxone while under general anesthesia (Loimer, Schmid, Presslich, & Lenz, 1988). Subsequent studies of this technique (O'Connor et al., 1998; Scherbaum et al., 1998) have used various approaches to detoxification and to sedation or general anesthesia. These studies have generally been small and methodologically limited, have not compared ultrarapid detoxification to other methods, and have provided little long-term follow-up (O'Connor & Kosten, 1998). In one study in which detoxified patients were followed up by telephone interview, only 10% continued naltrexone maintenance therapy for 7 months (Rabinowitz, Cohen, Tarrasch, & Kotler, 1997). Two studies have demonstrated that substantial withdrawal symptoms persist well beyond detoxification (Cucchia, Monnat, Spagnoli, Ferrero, & Bertschy, 1998; Scherbaum et al., 1998). In addition, the expense of this procedure (up to $7,500), the additional risk associated with general anesthesia, and safety concerns (San, Puig, Bulbena, & Farre, 1995; Pfab, Hirtl, & Zilker, 1999) limit its usefulness in clinical practice (O'Connor & Kosten, 1998). In at least one instance, safety concerns led to the termination of a clinical program that provided ultrarapid detoxification (Zielbauer, 1999). Thus, the widespread use of this procedure has been questioned (O'Connor & Kosten, 1998) and some authors have suggested that the procedure should be limited to clinical trials until its safety and efficacy can be further established (Strang, Bearn, & Gossop, 1997).

Opioid Detoxification in Physician Offices

At this point, opioid detoxification using opioid agonists is impractical in primary care settings given the lack of research on its effectiveness and the legal restrictions on use of opioid agonists for detoxification to inpatient settings and licensed treatment programs. However, detoxification with clonidine can be effective for some patients and may be feasible in the medical office setting

(O'Connor et al., 1997). This approach may be worth considering for highly motivated patients who have relatively low levels of dependence and who may not desire or need opioid agonist maintenance treatment. Although rapid opioid detoxification in primary care settings shows promise, more research is required before it can be generalized. Because this approach requires enhanced resources, it may be difficult for most physicians to perform. All patients who are being considered for detoxification should have a feasible and acceptable plan for immediate entry into postdetoxification substance abuse treatment.

PREVENTION OF RELAPSE BY USING MAINTENANCE MEDICATIONS

Although detoxification is a reasonable short-term approach designed to help selected patients achieve a drug-free state, long-term treatment is designed to prevent relapse to illicit drug use. Various pharmacologic therapies have been developed to promote abstinence from heroin, each designed to be administered in conjunction with counseling. The two pharmacologic strategies that have been developed are based on the use of an opioid antagonist or opioid agonists (Table 7.3).

Naltrexone

Opioid antagonists block opioid effects, thereby eliminating opioid-induced euphoria, diminishing the reinforcing effects of heroin (Rounsaville, 1995), and potentially extinguishing the association between conditioned stimuli and opioid use (Kieber, 1985). Opioid antagonists offer the advantage of treatment with medications that have no addictive potential or tolerance. Naltrexone, approved by the FDA in 1984, is the only opioid antagonist used for maintenance treatment of opioid dependence and is available in tablet form for use in

TABLE 7.3. Opioid Antagonists and Agonists Used to Treat Opioid Dependence

Medication	Action	Dose	Frequency	Availability
Naltrexone	Antagonist	50–100 mg orally	Daily or three times per week	Narcotic treatment program
Methadone	Agonist	20–100 mg orally	Daily	Narcotic treatment program
L-α acetylmethadol	Agonist	25–100 mg orally	Three times per week	Narcotic treatment program
Buprenorphine	Partial agonist	8–24 mg sublingually	Daily to three times per week	Pending approval by the Food and Drug Administration

detoxified patients. Naltrexone, a derivative of naloxone, displaces bound ago-nist (with receptor affinity 20 times that of morphine; Rounsaville, 1995) and blocks the effects of heroin administration (Kleber, 1985). Peak plasma con-centrations are achieved within 1 hour, and antagonist effects can last for up to 72 hours (Kleber, 1985). For example, dosages of 50, 100, and 150 mg/d can block the effect of 25 mg of intravenous heroin for 24, 48, and 72 hours, re-spectively (Kleber, 1985). Standard dosages of naltrexone are 50 mg/d or 100 mg on Monday and Wednesday and 150 mg on Friday (Farren, O'Malley, & Rounsaville, 1997). Naltrexone precipitates withdrawal in dependent patients who have not been abstinent for at least 7 days. In some patients, it may be necessary to document abstinence with urine toxicology or through a nalox-one challenge. Potential side effects of naltrexone include epigastric pain, nau-sea, headache, dizziness, nervousness, fatigue, or insomnia. Large dosages (up to 300 mg/d) may be hepatotoxic.

Despite the appealing properties of naltrexone, its clinical usefulness has been limited (Farren et al., 1997; Fram, Marmo, & Holden, 1989; Kosten, 1990; Rounsaville, 1995; Warner et al., 1997). Because naltrexone therapy requires abstinence, induction can be difficult and early dropout is common. In one treatment program, for example, only 15 of approximately 300 patients chose naltrexone instead of detoxification or methadone maintenance; of these 15, only 3 continued receiving therapy for more than 2 months (Fram et al., 1989). In another program, only 40% of 242 patients remained in treatment over 4 weeks (Greenstein, Arndt, McLellan, O'Brien, & Evans, 1984). Ran-domized trials have shown low retention rates (2%) (Clinical Evaluation, 1978) and no efficacy at reducing opioid use compared with placebo (San, Pomarol, Peri, Olie, & Cami, 1991). Naltrexone has shown some efficacy in the treat-ment of selected populations (for example, healthcare professionals; Ling & Wesson, 1984) and in combination with fluoxetine and weekly drug counsel-ing (Landabaso et al., 1998).

Methadone, L-α Acetylmethadol, and Buprenorphine

Recent research has demonstrated that repeated exposure to opioids, such as heroin, leads to changes in neurons in the locus ceruleus and mesolimbic areas of the brain and results in the clinical phenomena of tolerance, dependence, craving (Nestler & Aghajanian, 1997), and reward (Nestler, 1997). These neu-robiological changes provide insight into the chronic and relapsing nature of heroin dependence and a rationale for opioid agonist maintenance to stabilize these complex systems.

The primary goal of maintenance therapy is to prevent withdrawal and stabilize brain neurochemistry. This is accomplished by replacing heroin, a short-acting, euphorigenic opioid that is characterized by rapidly changing serum levels, with a long-acting, noneuphorigenic opioid that has relative steady-state pharmacokinetics. Opioid agonist maintenance therapies have several advantages over heroin. First, their slower onset of action minimizes their euphoric effect. Second, by occupying brain opioid receptors, they can block the euphoria associated with administration of heroin (competitive antagonism). Third, they eliminate the risk for infection associated with intravenous drug injection (O'Connor et al., 1994). Finally, opioid agonist maintenance prevents withdrawal (cross-tolerance) and thereby allows patients to function at a level that permits attention to the psychosocial aspects of treatment.

Methadone

Methadone hydrochloride, a synthetic, long-acting μ-opioid receptor agonist, is available in tablets or as a solution for oral or parenteral use in detoxification, maintenance, and treatment of severe pain. Peak blood levels after oral ingestion occur at 2 to 6 hours. Because of significant protein binding (> 90%), levels are constant over 24 hours. Methadone readily crosses the blood–brain barrier and undergoes extensive hepatic metabolism; urinary excretion is increased with acidification (Gilman, Goodman, Rall, & Murad, 1985). Methadone blocks many of the euphoric effects of exogenously administered opioids (Dole, Nyswander, & Kreek, 1966). However, when injected, methadone has potential for abuse in persons who are less opioid-dependent. Long-term treatment with methadone results in tolerance to its analgesic, sedative, and euphoric effects (Zweben & Payte, 1990), with minimal toxicity. Long-term side effects include constipation, weight gain, decreased libido, and menstrual irregularities (resulting from hyperprolactinemia). Methadone interacts with medications metabolized by the cytochrome P450 pathway, and plasma levels can be increased by concomitant administration of such medications as cimetidine, erythromycin, ketoconazole, and fluvoxamine (Kreek, 1986). Induction of hepatic microsomal enzymes leads to decreased plasma methadone levels and withdrawal due to interactions with alcohol, barbiturates, phenytoin, carbamazepine, isoniazid, rifampin (Kreek, 1986, 1988), retinovir (Iribarne, Berthou, et al., 1998), nevirapine (Altice, Friedland, & Cooney, 1999), and possibly efavirenz (Malaty & Kuper, 1999). Methadone is a racemic compound, and the D-isomer is an *N*-methyl-D-aspartate (NMDA)-receptor antagonist. Because of this property, it may be useful in patients with a high tolerance to opioids and in the management of neuropathic pain (Davis & Inturrisi, 1999; Ebert, Thorkildsen, Andersen, Christrup, & Hjeds, 1998; Gagnon & Bruera, 1999).

Current federal regulations mandate that methadone can be prescribed for detoxification or maintenance only by physicians with a special registration from the U.S. Drug Enforcement Administration (DEA; Cooper, 1995). This DEA registration is separate from the standard registration required for the prescription of controlled substances and is contingent upon compliance with DEA security regulations and other regulatory processes resulting from the Narcotic Addict Treatment Act of 1974 (Cooper, 1995).

The efficacy of methadone has been demonstrated empirically in several experimental and observational studies (Ball & Ross, 1991; Dole & Nyswander, 1965; Effective Medical Treatment, 1998; Gunne & Gronbladh, 1981; Newman, 1987; Newman & Whitehill, 1979). In one clinical trial of 169 persons seeking treatment for opioid dependence, opioid-positive results on urine toxicology tests decreased from 63% to 29% at 1-month follow-up in those randomly assigned to receive methadone. In contrast, a control group that remained on a waiting list for treatment had no change in their rate of opioid-positive urine test results (62% compared with 60% at 1 month; Yancovitz et al., 1991). An analysis of methadone maintenance by Ball and Ross (1991) involved 633 patients in six methadone treatment programs in New York, Philadelphia, and Baltimore. The prevalence of intravenous drug use decreased from 81% at admission to 29% at 4 years for the 388 patients who continued to receive treatment (Ball & Ross, 1991). Among the 105 patients who discontinued treatment, 82% resumed intravenous drug use by 12 months (Ball & Ross, 1991). These findings were recently replicated in the Drug Abuse Treatment Outcome Study (DATOS). In 727 patients who started methadone treatment, weekly heroin use dropped from 89% before treatment to 28% at 1 year (Hubbard, Craddock, Flynn, Anderson, & Etheridge, 1997).

In addition to decreasing heroin use, methadone maintenance has demonstrated other benefits (Effective Medical Treatment, 1998). In one study, criminal behavior measured as "crime days" per year decreased from a mean of 238 days before treatment to 32 days at 4 years of treatment (Ball & Ross, 1991). Similarly, the DATOS study showed a decrease in the number of patients who reported illegal activity (29% before treatment to 14% at 1-year follow-up; Hubbard et al., 1997). Methadone maintenance treatment has also been shown to reduce risk behavior for HIV infection and seroconversion in injection-drug users (Ball, Lange, Myers, & Friedman, 1988; Metzger et al., 1993; Metzger, Navaline, & Woody, 1998; Novick et al., 1990). For example, Metzger and colleagues demonstrated that HIV seroconversion occurred in 22% of 103 out-of-treatment patients compared with 3.5% of 152 patients receiving methadone maintenance (Metzger et al., 1993).

As seen with other medications, methadone dose can have a profound effect on therapeutic efficacy. The original study by Dole and Nyswander that demonstrated the efficacy of methadone in decreasing heroin use was conducted with daily doses ranging from 50 to 150 mg (Dole & Nyswander, 1965). Subsequently, several studies have demonstrated that higher doses of methadone (> 50 mg) are associated with better treatment retention and decreased illicit drug use (Caplehorn & Bell, 1991; Caplehorn, Bell, Kleinbaum, & Gebski, 1993; Strain, Bigelow, Liebson, & Stitzer, 1999; Strain, Stitzer, Liebson, & Bigelow, 1993). A recent trial noted lower rates of opioid-positive urine samples (53% compared with 62%; $P < 0.05$) in patients receiving 80 to 100 mg of methadone compared with those receiving 40 to 50 mg (Strain et al., 1999). However, because of misconceptions about the role of methadone dose (Cooper, 1992), many programs are reluctant to prescribe and patients are reluctant to take optimal doses. Thus, treatment practices and outcomes vary considerably (D'Aunno & Vaughn, 1992).

Methadone has been almost exclusively provided through narcotic treatment programs since 1972, when the FDA created regulations that specified the types and amount of treatment services to be provided (Ball & Ross, 1991). More than 900 programs currently exist in the United States, most in large cities. These programs usually have multidisciplinary staff who take a multilevel approach to determine frequency of program contact (daily compared with weekly) on the basis of federal regulations, duration of treatment, urine toxicology tests, patient compliance, and evidence of social stability.

Patient progress toward abstinence is monitored by patient self-report and assessment of results of urine toxicology tests. Continued illicit drug use is met with various strategies, including loss of privileges for take-home medication, increased frequency of clinic visits, and changes in medication dosage to combat withdrawal symptoms. Although evaluations of programs demonstrate continued illicit drug use in the overall client populations (Ball & Ross, 1991; D'Aunno & Vaughn, 1992), persistent drug use that does not respond to contingency management usually results in detoxification and program dismissal (Ball & Ross, 1991; D'Aunno & Vaughn, 1992; Ward, Mattick, & Hall, 1998).

L-α Acetylmethadol

L-α acetylmethadol (LAAM) is a long-acting derivative of methadone that was approved by the FDA for maintenance treatment in 1993. It is available in oral and parenteral form and is metabolized to more potent metabolites that have a prolonged duration of action. Peak blood levels are seen 4 to 8 hours after oral administration, and opioid withdrawal can be prevented for up to 72 hours (Blaine, 1978; Ling & Compton, 1997). This long duration of action makes it possible for patients to receive doses every 2 to 3 days, instead of daily as with methadone. Infrequent side effects noted with LAAM are similar to those seen with methadone.

Early work (Fraser & Isabell, 1952) helped to establish that LAAM was efficacious in preventing opioid withdrawal, and subsequent research provided evidence supporting the use of LAAM for opioid maintenance. These comparisons have demonstrated similar rates of retention in treatment (Freedman & Czertko, 1981; Jaffe et al., 1972; Ling, Charuvastra, Kaim, & Klett, 1976; Senay, Dorus, & Renault, 1977) and opioid-positive results on urine tests (Freedman & Czertko, 1981; Jaffe et al., 1970; Ling et al., 1976; Ling, Klett, & Gillis, 1978; Senay et al., 1977) in patients receiving methadone and LAAM. A recent meta-analysis of 14 randomized controlled trials comparing LAAM with methadone maintenance noted slightly greater treatment retention for methadone but a trend toward a greater decrease in illicit drug use with LAAM

(Glanz, Klawansky, McAuliffe, & Chalmers, 1997). Recent trials have demonstrated a dose-related decrease in heroin use in patients treated with LAAM (Eissenberg et al., 1997; Oliveto, Farren, & Kosten, 1998). For example, in one study, 180 patients were randomly assigned to receive LAAM 3 times per week: Monday, Wednesday, and Friday at 25, 25, and 35 mg; 50, 50, and 70 mg; and 100, 100, and 140 mg, respectively. Patients who received higher doses experienced more abstinence (Eissenberg et al., 1997).

Despite the advantages of LAAM, including more steady and sustained agonist activity than methadone, dosing three times per week, reduced dispensing costs, and decreased risk for diversion due to lack of "take-home" doses, a relatively small proportion of patients enrolled in opioid agonist maintenance receive it. In 1996, a survey found that only 62 of 750 treatment programs offered LAAM (Rawson, Hasson, Huber, McCann, & Ling, 1998). Reasons given for this slow acceptance were the additional state and local regulatory processes that are required, the reluctance of narcotic treatment programs to adopt new procedures, and the delay in insurance reimbursement (Rawson et al., 1998).

Buprenorphine

Buprenorphine hydrochloride, an investigational maintenance drug with unique pharmacologic properties, has not yet been approved for use as a maintenance medication but is being considered for approval by the FDA. If approved, buprenorphine, unlike methadone and LAAM, may be available outside of regulated narcotic treatment programs (Ling et al., 1998). Buprenorphine is a partial rather than full agonist at the μ-opioid receptor and a weak antagonist at the κ-receptor; thus, it may cause fewer withdrawal symptoms and have less potential for abuse, respiratory depression, and overdose (Bickel et al., 1988; Jasinski, Pevnick, & Griffith, 1978; Walsh, Preston, Stitzer, Cone, & Bigelow, 1994). In addition, buprenorphine has a slow rate of dissociation from opioid receptors, which results in a long duration of action.

Buprenorphine exists in parenteral form, a tablet for sublingual administration, and a new sublingual tablet that combines buprenorphine with naloxone. Buprenorphine is poorly absorbed through the gastrointestinal tract; however, sublingual administration results in plasma concentrations that are 60% to 70% of parenteral doses (Jasinski, Fudala, & Johnson, 1989). Constipation was the only significant side effect noted in a recent dose-ranging study of buprenorphine (Ling et al., 1998). Buprenorphine is metabolized by the cytochrome P450 pathway, and preliminary data suggest that potential drug-drug interactions exist between buprenorphine and benzodiazepines (Tracqui, Kintz, & Lundes, 1998), fluoxetine, fluvoxamine (Iribarne, Picart, Dreano, & Berthou, 1998), and ritonavir (Iribarne, Berthou, et al., 1998).

Jasinksi and coworkers (1978) established the opioid agonist effects of buprenorphine and its ability to block the effects of exogenous morphine administration. Subsequent research established its ability to suppress self-administration of heroin (Mello, Mendelson, & Kuehnle, 1982). Clinical trials have demonstrated the efficacy of buprenorphine over placebo in decreasing illicit opioid use (Johnson et al., 1995b) and have helped established the safety and efficacy of dosages ranging from 8 to 16 mg/d (Ling et al., 1998). In addition, it has been shown that daily and alternate-day buprenorphine dosing have equivalent effects on opioid withdrawal symptoms (Amass, Bickel, Higgins, & Badger, 1994; Fudala, Jaffe, Dax, & Johnson, 1990; Johnson et al., 1995a) and illicit opioid use (Johnson et al., 1995a). Administration three times per week also seems to be effective (O'Connor et al., 1998).

Clinical trials have shown that buprenorphine and low doses of methadone (20 to 30 mg) have similar effects on retention and illicit opioid use (Johnson, Jaffe, & Fudala, 1992; Ling, Wesson, Charuvastra, & Klett, 1996). Comparisons with higher doses of methadone (35 to 90 mg) have yielded inconclusive results; one trial demonstrated improved efficacy (Strain, Stitzer, Liebson, & Bigelow, 1994) and another demonstrated reduced efficacy (Kosten, Schottenfeld, Ziedonis, & Falcioni, 1993). Dose-ranging studies with buprenorphine have reported improved treatment outcomes with dosages of 6 to 16 mg/d compared with dosages of 1 to 4 mg/d (Ling et al., 1998; Kosten et al., 1993).

Nonpharmacologic Services for Opioid Agonist Maintenance

Nonpharmacologic or psychosocial counseling services are key components of the successful use of medications for opioid agonist maintenance. Psychosocial counseling services can vary by program and therapist (Ball & Ross, 1991; D'Aunno & Vaughn, 1992; Ward et al., 1998). Common components of individual counseling services include (a) addressing motivation for treatment, (b) teaching coping skills, (c) changing reinforcement contingencies, (d) fostering management of painful effects, (e) improving interpersonal functioning, and (f) fostering compliance with and retention in pharmacotherapy (Carroll & Schottenfeld, 1997). Although individual sessions are the hallmark of these services, narcotic treatment programs are often structured to provide other ancillary services, including group and family therapy, vocational counseling, case management, social service liaison, and education classes (Ball & Ross, 1991).

McLellan, Arndt, Metzger, Woody, and O'Brien (1993) demonstrated the importance of psychosocial counseling and ancillary services on treatment outcomes in methadone maintenance in a 6-month trial. New patients were randomly assigned to receive one of three levels of care: (a) methadone alone, (b) methadone plus standard counseling services, or (c) methadone and standard counseling services, plus on-site medical and psychiatric care, employment counseling, and family therapy services (McLellan et al., 1993). A dose-response effect was observed, and patients who received the standard or enhanced services had higher treatment retention rates than patients who received methadone alone. In addition, patients in the enhanced group had the fewest opiate-positive results on urine tests (McLellan et al., 1993). A cost-effectiveness analysis of these patients after 1 year showed that the annual cost per abstinent client was $16,485 for low levels of support, $9,804 for intermediate levels of support, and $11,818 for high levels of support (Kraft, Rothbard, Hadley, McLellan, & Asch, 1997).

The duration of opioid agonist maintenance varies substantially according to patient characteristics. A recent national survey of methadone treatment programs demonstrated that 58% of programs encouraged their clients to undergo detoxification within 3 to 12 months of admission and that the average length of treatment was 20 months (D'Aunno & Vaughn, 1992). However, on the basis of the high rates of relapse observed in detoxified patients (Ball & Ross, 1991; Strain et al., 1993) and the risk for complications resulting from relapse (Stein, 1990), some authorities advocate a policy of providing treatment as long as treatment is clinically indicated and the patient continues to benefit from treatment, wishes to remain in treatment, remains at risk for relapse to heroin use, and has no significant side effects (Payte & Khuri, 1993).

Opioid Maintenance in Physician Offices

Because of the success of long-term methadone treatment of opioid-dependent patients and growing evidence that primary care physicians can play a major role in treating alcohol problems (Fleming, Barry, Maxwell, Johnson, & London, 1997) and possibly heroin dependence (O'Connor et al., 1998), interest has increased in providing ongoing opioid maintenance therapy from physicians' offices (Cooper, 1995; Novick et al., 1988, 1994). "Medical maintenance" is defined by Novick and colleagues (1988) as the treatment by primary care physicians of rehabilitated methadone maintenance recipients who are stable and employed, are not abusing drugs, and do not need supportive services. The potential advantages of medical maintenance include the ability to expand opioid maintenance treatment capacity and a recognition of the view that for some patients, opioid dependence is a chronic disease with a persistent neurochemical disorder (Dole, 1988). In addition, there is a desire to allocate traditional drug treatment services more appropriately and to increase the number of practicing physicians involved in the care of opioid-dependent patients (Cooper, 1995; Effective Medical Treatment, 1998). Finally, the physician's office may provide treatment in a setting that minimizes the stigma of drug treatment programs and limits contact with drug-using patients.

Published reports of two successful medical maintenance programs support the idea of transferring the care of stabilized, methadone-maintained patients to these settings (Novick et al., 1988, 1994; Senay et al., 1993). One program in New York City reported 85% retention at 3 years in 100 patients whose care was transferred from conventional methadone maintenance treatment to medical maintenance (Novick et al., 1994). A randomized clinical trial compared medical maintenance with maintenance in a methadone program and reported 1-year retention rates of 73% for patients in both groups (Senay et al., 1993). Of interest, a recent clinical trial showed improved retention and decreased illicit opioid use when buprenorphine was administered three times per week in a primary care setting compared with thrice-weekly buprenorphine maintenance in a formal drug treatment program (O'Connor et al., 1998).

An important unanswered question about medical maintenance is patient selection. Previous programs (Novick et al., 1988; 1994; Senay et al., 1993) have used patient factors, including longer duration of methadone maintenance without relapse, stable means of financial support, absence of concurrent substance abuse or dependence, absence of substantial untreated comorbid psychiatric disease, and patient motivation to participate, to identify successful patients for medical maintenance. Of note, the duration of ongoing methadone maintenance required before eligibility for medical maintenance has varied between 5 years (Novick et al., 1988, 1994) and 1 year (Senay et al., 1993). In contrast, in a study that examined the efficacy of buprenorphine in a primary care setting, some enrolled patients were not receiving any treatment at the time of enrollment (O'Connor et al., 1998).

Medical maintenance pilot programs are underway in Connecticut, Maryland, New York, and Washington State. Results from these efforts are expected to inform decisions regarding types of patients, physician training, and the role of the treatment program. In these programs, the traditional treatment program serves as the "hub" and the physician's offices represent "spokes" of a wheel. Therefore, patients receiving medical maintenance remain registered in their treatment program and the medical maintenance physicians are enrolled as medical staff in that program; this can facilitate transfer of the patient to the hub program in the event of a substantial relapse. The success of the early models of medical maintenance has resulted in a call for the expansion of these programs. A recent survey found that 30 state authorities favored off-site physician linkages with methadone programs as an adjunct to traditional methadone maintenance treatment (Parrino, 1998). Until the models for these programs are fully developed and the legal restrictions on them are changed, office-based opioid maintenance will not be feasible. However, recent initiatives in office-based maintenance are promising and may be feasible soon.

MATCHING PHARMACOLOGIC APPROACHES TO PATIENTS WITH HEROIN DEPENDENCE

The choice between detoxification and opioid agonist therapy for pharmacologic management of heroin-dependent patients can be difficult, and no clear guidelines exist. Federal requirements have evolved from the fairly restrictive criteria that were in place when methadone was introduced in the 1960s (State Methadone Treatment Guidelines, 1993). Initially, candidates for methadone maintenance were required to be 21 to 40 years of age, to have been addicted to heroin for at least 4 years, to have evidence of relapse with previous attempts at detoxification, and to have no major medical or psychiatric problems or polysubstance abuse. Pregnant women were not eligible. Current criteria for maintenance with methadone or LAAM specify that patients must be at least 18 years of age and have at least a 1-year history of opioid addiction and evidence of physiologic dependence (State, 1993). Medical, psychiatric, or comorbid substance use disorders do not indicate obligatory exclusion, and pregnant women can be admitted under modified criteria (for example, heroin dependence less than 1 year with current use; State, 1993).

These regulations notwithstanding, the decision to institute opioid agonist maintenance involves a careful consideration of clinical characteristics and an evaluation of the risks and benefits for an individual patient. For example, an attempt at detoxification would be an appropriate first choice of treatment for a patient with a low level of heroin use, few symptoms of dependence, and no substantial risk for acquiring or transmitting bloodborne infections (for example, through intranasal heroin use). However, for patients with a long history of dependence, previous failed attempts at detoxification, high levels of heroin use, and substantial risk for infectious complications (for example, injection drug use or seropositive HIV status), opioid agonist or partial agonist maintenance is likely to be more effective in reducing the harm associated with heroin use and in promoting abstinence. Clearly, further research on the differential roles of detoxification and maintenance therapies is needed to identify the most appropriate strategies to match patient to treatment.

SUMMARY: THE ROLES OF PHYSICIANS IN THE MANAGEMENT OF HEROIN-DEPENDENT PATIENTS

Patients who are dependent on heroin or other illicit drugs provide unique challenges for physicians. Because heroin dependence has major medical sequelae, patients are likely to interact with various aspects of the healthcare system, including the emergency department, hospital, and physician's office. Physicians in these settings therefore need to be able to take an active role in the identification and management of patients with drug problems if they are to provide effective and efficient healthcare.

The major roles for physicians in managing heroin-dependent patients and patients who use other substances include universal screening for substance use, assessing patients for health and behavioral problems related to substance use, and providing appropriate preventive health services. In addition, physicians should be able to provide an appropriate level of advice and counseling and refer patients to appropriate specialty services for treatment of

TABLE 7.4. Additional Resources for Treatment of Opioid Dependence

A Guide to Substance Abuse Services for Primary Care Clinicians. Rockville, MD: U.S. Department of Health and Human Services, Public Health Service, Substance Abuse and Mental Health Services Administration, Center for Substance Abuse Treatment; 1997. Treatment Improvement Protocol Series, no. 24

Effective Medical Treatment of Opiate Addiction. National Institute of Health Consensus Statement. 1997; 15:1–41.

The National Institute on Drug Abuse (http://www.nida.hih.gov)

drug dependence. Because these patients often present with a diverse set of needs, careful coordination with physicians and professionals from other disciplines is usually necessary. Despite these complexities, internists and other primary care physicians are well suited to provide longitudinal care for heroin-dependent patients. Additional resources on treatment of opioid dependence can be found in Table 7.4.

Ongoing and future research promises to further unravel the mysteries of drug dependence and provide new insights into patient management. New treatment approaches are constantly being evaluated and developed. Opioid maintenance treatment has been particularly successful in this regard, and new approaches to patient-treatment matching are under evaluation. Office-based treatment strategies may increase access to maintenance treatment while greatly expanding the role of internists and other physicians in patient management. Although prevention of drug abuse is a new science that holds promise for the future, recognition and treatment of drug abuse are essential given the impact of opioid dependence on individual persons and on society.

REFERENCES

Altice, F. L., Friedland, G. H., & Cooney, E. L. (1999). Nevirapine induced opiate withdrawal among injection drug users with HIV infection receiving methadone. *AIDS, 13,* 957–962.

Amass, L., Bickel, W. K., Higgins, S. T., & Badger, G. J. (1994). Alternate-day dosing during buprenorphine treatment of opioid dependence. *Life Sciences, 54,* 1215–1228.

Amass, L., Bickel, W. K., Higgins, S. T., & Hughes, J. R. (1994). A preliminary investigation of outcome following gradual or rapid buprenorphine detoxification. *Journal of Addictive Disorders, 13,* 33–45.

American Psychiatric Association. (1994). *Diagnostic and statistical manual of mental disorders* (4th ed.). Washington, DC: Author.

Ball, J. C., Lange, W. R., Myers, C. P., & Friedman, S. R. (1988). Reducing the risk of AIDS through methadone maintenance treatment. *Journal of Health and Social Behavior, 29,* 214–226.

Ball, J. C., & Ross, A. (1991). *The effectiveness of methadone maintenance treatment: Patients, programs, services, and outcomes.* New York: Springer-Verlag.

Bearn, J., Gossop, M., & Strang, J. (1996). Randomised double-blind comparison of lofexidine and methadone in the in-patient treatment of opiate withdrawal. *Drug and Alcohol Dependence, 43,* 87–91.

Bearn, J., Gossop, M., & Strang, J. (1998). Accelerated lofexidine treatment regimen compared with conventional lofexidine and methadone treatment for in-patient opiate detoxification. *Drug and Alcohol Dependence, 50,* 227–232.

Bickel, W. K., Stitzer, M. L., Bigelow, G. E., Liebson, I. A., Jasinski, D. R., & Johnson, R. E. (1988). A clinical trial of buprenorphine: Comparison with methadone in the detoxification of heroin addicts. *Clinical Pharmacology and Therapy, 43,* 72–78.

Blaine, J. D. (1978). Early clinical studies of levo-alpha acetylmethadol (LAAM): An opiate for use in the medical treatment of chronic heroin dependence. *NIDA Research Monograph, 19,* 249–259.

Brewer, D. D., Fleming, C. B., Haggerty, K. P., & Catalano, R. F. (1998). Drug use predictors of partner violence in opiate-dependent women. *Violence and Victims, 13,* 107–115.

Brooner, R. K., King, V. L., Kidorf, M., Schmidt, C. W. Jr., & Bigelow, G. E. (1997). Psychiatric and substance use comorbidity among treatment-seeking opioid abusers. *Archives of General Psychiatry, 54,* 71–80.

Caplehorn, J. R., & Bell, J. (1991). Methadone dosage and retention of patients in maintenance treatment. *Medical Journal of Australia, 154,* 195–199.

Caplehorn, J. R., Bell, J., Kleinbaum, D. G., & Gebski, V. J. (1993). Methadone dose and heroin use during maintenance treatment. *Addiction, 88,* 119–124.

Carroll, K. M., & Schottenfeld, R. (1997). Nonpharmacologic approaches to substance abuse treatment. *Medical Clinics of North America, 81,* 927–944.

Charney, D. S., Heninger, G. R., & Kleber, H. D. (1986). The combined use of clonidine and naltrexone as a rapid, safe, and effective treatment of abrupt withdrawal from methadone. *American Journal of Psychiatry, 143,* 831–837.

Charney, D. S., Sternberg, D. E., Kleber, H. D., Heninger, G. R., & Redmond, D. E., Jr. (1981). The clinical use of clonidine in abrupt withdrawal from methadone. Effects on blood pressure and specific signs and symptoms. *Archives of General Psychiatry, 38,* 1273–1277.

Cherubin, C. E, & Sapira, J. D. (1993). The medical complications of drug addiction and the medical assessment of the intravenous drug user: 25 years later. *Annals of Internal Medicine, 119,* 1017–1028.

Cheskin, L. J., Fudala, P. J., & Johnson, R. E. (1994). A controlled comparison of buprenorphine and clonidine for acute detoxification from opioids. *Drug and Alcohol Dependence, 36,* 115–121.

Chutuape, M. A., Brooner, R. K., & Stitzer, M. (1997). Sedative use disorders in opiate-dependent patients: Association with psychiatric and other substance use disorders. *Journal of Nervous and Mental Disorders, 185,* 289–297.

Clinical evaluation of naltrexone treatment of opiate-dependent individuals. (1978). Report of the National Research Council Committee on Clinical Evaluation of Narcotic Antagonists. *Archives of General Psychiatry, 35,* 335–340.

Cooper, J. R. (1992). Ineffective use of psychoactive drugs. Methadone treatment is no exception. *Journal of the American Medical Association, 267,* 281–282.

Cooper, J. R. (1995). Including narcotic addiction treatment in an office-based practice. *Journal of the American Medical Association, 273,* 1619–1620.

Cucchia, A. T., Monnat, M., Spagnoli, J., Ferrero, F., & Bertschy, G. (1998). Ultra-rapid opiate detoxification using deep sedation with oral midazolam: Short and long-term results. *Drug and Alcohol Dependence, 52,* 243–250.

Darke, S., & Ross, J. (1997). Polydrug dependence and psychiatric comorbidity among heroin injectors. *Drug and Alcohol Dependence, 48,* 135–141.

Dashe, J. S., Jackson, G. L., Olscher, D. A., Zane, E. H., & Wendel, G. D., Jr. (1998).

Opioid detoxification in pregnancy. *Obstetrics and Gynecology, 92,* 854–858.

D'Aunno, T., & Vaughn, T. E. (1992). Variations in methadone treatment practices. Results from a national study. *Journal of the American Medical Association, 267,* 253–258.

Davis, A. M, & Inturrisi, C. E. (1999). D-Methadone blocks morphine tolerance and *N*-methyl-D-aspartate-induced hyperalgesia. *Journal of Pharmacology and Experimental Therapeutics, 289,* 1048–1053.

Dole, V. P. (1988). Implications of methadone maintenance for theories of narcotic addiction. *Journal of the American Medical Association, 260,* 3025–3029.

Dole, V. P., & Nyswander, M. (1965). A medical treatment for diacetylmorphine (heroin) addiction. A clinical trial with methadone hydrochloride. *Journal of the American Medical Association, 193,* 646–650.

Dole, V. P., Nyswander, M. E., & Kreek, M. J. (1966). Narcotic blockade. *Archives of Internal Medicine, 118,* 304–309.

Drug Abuse Warning Network. (1996). *Year-end preliminary estimates.* Rockville, MD: Office of Applied Studies, Department of Health and Human Services, Substance Abuse and Mental Health Services Administration.

Ebert, B., Thorkildsen, C., Andersen, S., Christrup, L. L., & Hjeds, H. (1998). Opioid analgesics as noncompetitive *N*-methyl-D-aspartate (NMDA) antagonists. *Biochemical Pharmacology, 56,* 553–559.

Effective medical treatment of opiate addiction. (1998). National Consensus Development Panel on Effective Medical Treatment of Opiate Addiction. *Journal of the American Medical Association, 280,* 1936–1943.

Eissenberg, T., Bigelow, G. E., Strain, E. C., Walsh, S. L., Brooner, R. K., Stitzer, M. L., et al. (1997). Dose-related efficacy of levomethadyl acetate for treatment of opioid dependence. A randomized clinical trial. *Journal of the American Medical Association, 277,* 1945–1951.

Farren, C. K., O'Malley, S., & Rounsaville, B. (1997). Naltrexone and opiate abuse. In S. M. Stine & T. R. Kosten (Eds.), *New treatments for opiate dependence* (pp. 104–123). New York: Guilford.

Fleming, M. F., Barry, K. L., Manwell, L. B., Johnson, K., & London, R. (1997). Brief physician advice for problem alcohol drinkers. A randomized controlled trial in community-based primary care practices. *Journal of the American Medical Association, 277,* 1039–1045.

Fram, D. H., Marmo, J., & Holden, R. Naltrexone treatment—the problem of patient acceptance. *Journal of Substance Abuse Treatment, 6,* 119–122.

Fraser, H. F., & Isbell, H. (1952). Actions and addiction liabilities of alpha-acetylmethadols in man. *Journal of Pharmacology and Experimental Therapeutics, 105,* 458–465.

Freedman, R. R., & Czertko, G. (1981). A comparison of thrice weekly LAAM and daily methadone in employed heroin addicts. *Drug and Alcohol Dependence, 8,* 215–222.

Friedmann, P. D., Saitz, R., & Samet, J. H. (1998). Management of adults recovering from alcohol or other drug problems: Relapse prevention in primary care. *Journal of the American Medical Association, 279,* 1227–1231.

Fudala, P. J., Jaffe, J. H., Dax, E. M., & Johnson, R. E. (1990). Use of buprenorphine in the treatment of opioid addiction. II. Physiologic and behavioral effects of daily and alternate-day administration and abrupt withdrawal. *Clinical Pharmacology and Therapeutics, 47,* 525–534.

Fultz, J. M., & Senay, E. C. (1975). Guidelines for the management of hospitalized narcotics addicts. *Annals of Internal Medicine, 82,* 815–818.

Gagnon, B., & Bruera, E. (1999). Differences in the ratios of morphine to methadone in patients with neuropathic pain versus non-neuropathic pain. *Journal of Pain and*

Symptom Management, 18, 120–125.

Gilman, A. G., Goodman, L. S., Rall, T. W., & Murad, F., (Eds.). (1985). *Goodman and Gilman's the pharmacologic basis of therapeutics* (7th ed.). New York: Macmillan.

Glanz, M., Klawansky, S., McAullife, W., & Chalmers, T. (1997). Methadone vs. L-alpha-acetylmethadol (LAAM) in the treatment of opiate addiction. A meta-analysis of the randomized, controlled trials. *The American Journal on Addiction, 6,* 339–349.

Gossop, M. (1988). Clonidine and the treatment of the opiate withdrawal syndrome. *Drug and Alcohol Dependence, 21,* 253–259.

Gossop, M. (1990). The development of a Short Opiate Withdrawal Scale (SOWS). *Addictive Behaviors, 15,* 487–490.

Greenstein, R. A., Arndt, I. C., McLellan, A. T., O'Brien, C. P., & Evans, B. (1984). Naltrexone: A clinical perspective. *Journal of Clinical Psychiatry, 45*(9, Pt. 2), 25–28.

Gunne, L. M, & Gronbladh, L. (1981). The Swedish methadone maintenance program: A controlled study. *Drug and Alcohol Dependence, 7,* 249–256.

Hamid, A., Curtis, R., McCoy, K., McGuire, J., Conde, A., Bushell, W., et al. (1997). The heroin epidemic in New York City: Current status and prognoses. *Journal of Psychoactive Drugs, 29,* 375–391.

Harwood, H. J., Fountain, D., & Livermore, G. (1998). *The economic costs of alcohol and drug abuse in the United States, 1992.* The Lewin Group. Rockville, MD: National Institute on Drug Abuse.

Hubbard, R. L., Craddock, S. G., Flynn, P. M., Anderson, J., & Etheridge, R. M. (1997). Overview of 1-year follow-up outcomes in the Drug Abuse Treatment Outcome Study (DATOS). *Psychology of Addictive Behaviors, 11,* 261–278.

Iribarne, C., Berthou, F., Carihant, D., Dreano, Y., Picart, D., Lohezic, F., et al. (1998). Inhibition of methadone and buprenorphine *N*-dealkylations by three HIV-1 protease inhibitors. *Drug Metabolism and Disposition, 26,* 257–260.

Iribarne, C., Picart, D., Dreano, Y., & Berthou, F. (1998). In vitro interactions between fluoxetine or fluvoxamine and methadone or buprenorphine. *Fundamental Clinical Pharmacology, 12,* 194–199.

Jaffe, J. H., Schuster, C. R., Smith, B. B., & Blachley, P. H. (1970). Comparison of acetylmethadol and methadone in the treatment of long-term heroin users. A pilot study. *Journal of the American Medical Association, 211,* 1834–1836.

Jaffe, J. H., Senay, E. C., Schuster, C. R., Renault, P. R., Smith, B., & DiMenza, S. (1972). Methadyl acetate vs methadone. A double-blind study in heroin users. *Journal of the American Medical Association, 222,* 437–442.

Jasinski, D. R., Fudala, P. J., & Johnson, R. E. (1989). Sublingual versus subcutaneous buprenorphine in opiate abusers. *Clinical Pharmacology and Therapeutics, 45,* 513–519.

Jasinski, D. R., Pevnick, J. S., & Griffith, J. D. (1978). Human pharmacology and abuse potential of the analgesic buprenorphine. A potential agent for treating narcotic addiction. *Archives of General Psychiatry, 35,* 501–516.

Johnson, R. E., Eissenberg, T., Stitzer, M. L., Strain, E. C., Liebson, I. A., & Bigelow, G. E. (1995). A placebo controlled clinical trial of buprenorphine as a treatment for opioid dependence. *Drug and Alcohol Dependence, 40,* 17–25.

Johnson, R. E., Eissenberg, T., Stitzer, M. L., Strain, E. C., Liebson, I. A., & Bigelow, G. E. (1995). Buprenorphine treatment of opioid dependence: Clinical trial of daily versus alternate-day dosing. *Drug and Alcohol Dependence, 40,* 27–35.

Johnson, R. E., Jaffe, J. H., & Fudala, P. J. (1992). A controlled trial of buprenorphine treatment for opioid dependence. *Journal of the American Medical Association, 267,* 2750–2755.

Kahn, A., Mumford, J. P., Rogers, G. A., & Beckford, H. (1997). Double-blind study of lofexidine and clonidine in the detoxification of opiate addicts in hospital. *Drug and Alcohol Dependence, 44,* 57–61.

Kleber, H. D. (1985). Naltrexone. *Journal of Substance Abuse Treatment, 2,* 117–122.

Kleber, H. D., Riordan, C. E., Rounsaville, B., Kosten, T., Charney, D., Gaspari, J., et al. (1985). Clonidine in outpatient detoxification from methadone maintenance. *Archives of General Psychiatry, 42,* 391–394.

Kleber, H. D., Topazian, M., Gaspari, J., Riordan, C. E., & Kosten, T. (1987). Clonidine and naltrexone in the outpatient treatment of heroin withdrawal. *American Journal of Drug and Alcohol Abuse, 13,* 1–17.

Kosten, T. R. (1990). Current pharmacotherapies for opioid dependence. *Psychopharmacology Bulletin, 26,* 69–74.

Kosten, T. R., & McCance, E. (1996). A review of pharmacotherapies for substance abuse. *The American Journal on Addiction, 5,* 58–65.

Kosten, T. R., Schottenfeld, R., Ziedonis, D., & Falcioni, J. (1993). Buprenorphine versus methadone maintenance for opioid dependence. *Journal of Nervous and Mental Disease, 181,* 358–364.

Kraft, K. M., Rothbard, A. B., Hadley, T. R., McLelian, A. T., & Asch, D. A. (1997). Are supplementary services provided during methadone maintenance really cost-effective? *American Journal of Psychiatry, 154,* 1214–1219.

Kreek, M. J. (1986). Drug interactions with methadone in humans. *NIDA Research Monograph, 68,* 193–225.

Kreek, M. J. (1988). Opiate-ethanol interactions: Implications for the biological basis and treatment of combined addictive diseases. *NIDA Research Monograph, 81,* 428–439.

Landabaso, M. A., Iraurgi, I., Jimenez-Lerma, J. M., Sanz, J., Fernandez De Corres, B., Araluce, K., et al. (1998). A randomized trial of adding fluoxetine to a naltrexone treatment programme for heroin addicts. *Addiction, 93,* 739–744.

Liebschutz, J. M., Mulvey, K. P., & Samet, J. H. (1997). Victimization among substance-abusing women. Worse health outcomes. *Archives of Internal Medicine, 157,* 1093–1097.

Lin, S. K., Strang, J., Su, L. W., Tsai, C. J., & Hu, W. H. (1997). Double-blind randomised controlled trial of lofexidine versus clonidine in the treatment of heroin withdrawal. *Drug and Alcohol Dependence, 48,* 127–133.

Ling, W., Charuvastra, C., Collins, J. F., Batki, S., Brown, L. S., Jr., Kintaudi, P., et al. (1998). Buprenorphine maintenance treatment of opiate dependence: A multicenter, randomized clinical trial. *Addiction, 93,* 475–486.

Ling, W., Charuvastra, C., Kaim, S. C., & Klett, C. J. (1976). Methadyl acetate and methadone as maintenance treatments for heroin addicts. A veterans administration cooperative study. *Archives of General Psychiatry, 33,* 709–720.

Ling, W., & Compton, P. (1997). Opiate maintenance therapy with LAAM. In S. M. Stine & T. R. Kosten (Eds.), *New treatments for opiate dependence* (pp. 286). New York: Guilford.

Ling, W., Kilett, C. J., & Gillis, R. D. (1978). A cooperative clinical study of methadyl acetate. I. Three-time-a-week regimen. *Archives of General Psychiatry, 35,* 345–353.

Ling, W., & Wesson, D. R. (1984). Naltrexone treatment for addicted health-care professionals: A collaborative private practice experience. *Journal of Clinical Psychiatry, 45*(9, Pt. 2), 46–48.

Ling, W., Wesson, D. R., Charuvastra, C., & Klett, C. J. (1996). A controlled trial comparing buprenorphine and methadone maintenance in opioid dependence. *Archives of General Psychiatry, 53,* 401–407.

Loimer, N., Schmid, R., Presslich, O., & Lenz, K. (1988). Naloxone treatment for opiate withdrawal syndrome. *British Journal of Psychiatry, 153,* 851–852.

Malaty, L. I., & Kuper, J. J. (1999). Drug interactions of HIV protease inhibitors. *Drug Safety, 20,* 147–169.

McCann, M. J., Miotto, K., Rawson, R. A., Huber, A., Shoptaw, S., & Ling, W. (1997). Outpatient non-opioid detoxification for opioid withdrawal. Who is likely to benefit? *American Journal of Addiction, 6,* 218–223.

McLellan, A. T., Arndt, I. O., Metzger, D. S., Woody, G. E., & O'Brien, C. P. (1993). The effects of psychosocial services in substance abuse treatment. *Journal of the American Medical Association, 69,* 1953–1959.

Mello, N. K., Mendelson, J. H., & Kuehnie, J. C. (1982). Buprenorphine effects on human heroin self-administration: An operant analysis. *Journal of Pharmacology and Experimental Therapeutics, 223,* 30–39.

Metzger, D. S., Navaline, H., & Woody, G. E. (1998). Drug abuse treatment as AIDS prevention. *Public Health Report, 113*(Suppl. 1), 97–106.

Metzger, D. S., Woody, G. E., McLellan, A. T., O'Brien, C. P., Druley, P., Navaline, H., et al. (1993). Human immunodeficiency virus seroconversion among intravenous drug users in- and out-of-treatment: An 18-month prospective follow-up. *Journal of Acquired Immune Deficiency Syndromes, 6,* 1049–1056.

National Household Survey on Drug Abuse. (1999). *Main findings, 1997.* Rockville, MD: U.S. Department of Health and Human Services, Public Health Service, Alcohol, Drug Abuse, and Mental Health Services Administration.

Nestler, E. J. (1997). Basic neurobiology of opiate addiction. In S. M. Stine & T. R. Kosten (Eds.), *New treatments for opiate dependence* (p. 286). New York: Guilford.

Nestler, E. J., & Aghajanian, G. K. (1997). Molecular and cellular basis of addiction. *Science, 278,* 58–63.

Newman, R. G., & Whitehill, W. B. (1979). Double-blind comparison of methadone and placebo maintenance treatments of narcotic addicts in Hong Kong. *Lancet, 2,* 485–488.

Newman, R. G. (1987). Methadone treatment. Defining and evaluating success. *New England Journal of Medicine, 317,* 447–450.

Nigam, A. K., Ray, R., & Tripathi, B. M. (1993). Buprenorphine in opiate withdrawal: A comparison with clonidine. *Journal of Substance and Abuse Treatment, 10,* 391–394.

Novick, D. M, Joseph, H., Croxson, T. S., Salsitz, E. A., Wang, G., Richman, B. L., et al. (1990). Absence of antibody to human immunodeficiency virus in long-term, socially rehabilitated methadone maintenance patients. *Archives of Internal Medicine, 150,* 97–99.

Novick, D. M., Joseph, H., Salsitz, E. A., Kalin, M. F., Keefe, J. B., Miller, E. L., et al. (1994). Outcomes of treatment of socially rehabilitated methadone maintenance patients in physicians' offices (medical maintenance): Follow-up at three and a half to nine and a fourth years. *Journal of General Internal Medicine, 9,* 127–130.

Novick, D. M., Pascarelli, E. F., Joseph, H., Salsitz, E. A., Richman, B. L., Des Jarlais, D. C., et al. (1988). Methadone maintenance patients in general medical practice. A preliminary report. *Journal of the American Medical Association, 259,* 3299–3302.

O'Connor, P. G., Selwyn, P. A.,& Schottenfeld, R. S. (1994). Medical care for injection drug users with human immunodeficiency virus infection. *New England Journal of Medicine, 331,* 450–459.

O'Connor, P. G., Waugh, M. E., Carroll, K. M., Rounsaville, B. J., Diagkogiannis, I. A., & Schottenfeld, R. S. (1995). Primary care-based ambulatory opioid detoxification: The results of a clinical trial. *Journal of General Internal Medicine, 10,* 255–260.

O'Connor, P. G., Carroll, K. M., Shi, J. M., Schottenfeld, R. S., Kosten, T. R., & Rounsaville, B. J. (1997). Three methods of opioid detoxification in a primary care setting. A randomized trial. *Annals of Internal Medicine, 127,* 526–530.

O'Connor, P. G., & Kosten, T. R. (1998). Rapid and ultrarapid opioid detoxification techniques. *Journal of the American Medical Association, 279,* 229–234.

O'Connor, P. G., Oliveto, A. H., Shi, J. M., Triffieman, E. G., Carroll, K. M., Kosten, T. R., et al. (1998). A randomized trial of buprenorphine maintenance for heroin dependence in a primary care clinic for substance users versus a methadone clinic. *American Journal of Medicine, 105,* 100–105.

Oliveto, A. H., Farren, C., & Kosten, T. R. (1998). Effect of LAAM dose on opiate use in opioid-dependent patients. A pilot study. *The American Journal on Addictions, 7,* 272–282.

Parrino, M. W. (1998). The tornado of change. *Journal of Maintenance in the Addictions, 1,* 71–80.

Payte, J. T., & Khuri, E. T. (1993). *Treatment duration and patient retention.* Report no. 93–1991. Center for Substance Abuse Treatment. Rockville, MD: U.S. Department of Health and Human Services.

Pfab, R., Hirti, C., & Zilker, T. (1999). Opiate detoxification under anesthesia: No apparent benefit but suppression of thyroid hormones and risk of pulmonary and renal failure. *Journal of Toxicology Clinical Toxicology, 37,* 43–50.

Prochaska, J. O., DiClemente, C. C., Velicer, W. F., & Rossi, J. S. (1992). Criticisms and concerns of the transtheoretical model in light of recent research. *British Journal of Addiction, 87,* 825–828; discussion 833–835.

Rabinowitz, J., Cohen, H., Tarrasch, R., & Kotler, M. (1997). Compliance to naltrexone treatment after ultra-rapid opiate detoxification: An open label naturalistic study. *Drug and Alcohol Dependence, 47,* 77–86.

Rawson, R. A., Hasson, A. L., Huber, A. M., McCann, M. J., & Ling, W. (1998). A 3-year progress report on the implementation of LAAM in the United States. *Addiction, 93,* 533–540.

Regidor, E., Barrio, G., de la Fuente, L., & Rodriguez, C. (1996). Non-fatal injuries and the use of psychoactive drugs among young adults in Spain. *Drug and Alcohol Dependence, 40,* 249–259.

Resnick, R. B., Kestenbaum, R. S., Washton, A., & Poole, D. (1977) Naloxone-precipitated withdrawal: A method for rapid induction onto naltrexone. *Clinical and Pharmacology Therapy, 21,* 409–413.

Rosen, M. I., McMahon, T. J., Hameedi, F. A., Pearsall, H. R., Woods, S. W., Kreek, M. J., et al. (1996). Effect of clonidine pretreatment on naloxone-precipitated opiate withdrawal. *Journal of Pharmacology and Experimental Therapeutics, 276,* 1128–1135.

Rounsaville, B. J. (1995). Can psychotherapy rescue naltrexone treatment of opioid addiction? *NIDA Research Monograph, 150,* 37–52.

Samet, J. H., Rollinick, S., & Barnes, H. (1996). Beyond CAGE. A brief clinical approach after detection of substance abuse. *Archives of Internal Medicine, 156,* 2287–2293.

Samet, J. H., & O'Connor, P. G. (1998). Alcohol abusers in primary care: Readiness to change behavior. *American Journal of Medicine, 105,* 302–306.

San, L., Pomaroi, G., Peri, J. M., Olie, J. M., & Cami, J. (1991). Follow-up after a six-month maintenance period on naltrexone versus placebo in heroin addicts. *British Journal of Addiction, 86,* 983–990.

San, L., Puig, M., Bulbena, A., & Farre, M. (1995). High risk of ultrashort noninvasive opiate detoxification [Letter]. *American Journal of Psychiatry, 152,* 956.

Scherbaum, N., Klein, S., Kaube, H., Kienbaum, P., Peters, J., & Gastpar, M. (1998). Alternative strategies of opiate detoxification: Evaluation of the so-called ultra-rapid detoxification. *Pharmacopsychiatry, 31,* 205–209.

Schorling, J. B., & Buchsbaum, D. (1997). Screening for alcohol and drug abuse. *Medical Clinics of North America, 81,* 845–865.

Schottenfeld, R. S., O'Malley, S., Abdul-Salaam, K., & O'Connor, P. G. (1993). Decline in intravenous drug use among treatment-seeking opiate users. *Journal of Substance Abuse Treatment, 10,* 5–10.

Senay, E. C., Barthwell, A. G., Marks, R., Bokos, P., Gillman, D., White, R. (1993). Medical maintenance: A pilot study. *Journal of Addictive Diseases, 12,* 59–76.

Senay, E. C., Dorus, W., & Renault, P. F. (1977). Methadyl acetate and methadone. An open comparison. *Journal of the American Medical Association, 237,* 138–142.

Sporer, K. A. (1999). Acute heroin overdose. *Annals of Internal Medicine, 130,* 584–590.

State Methadone Treatment Guidelines. Vol. 1. (1993). Rockville, MD: U.S. Department of Health and Human Services.

Stein, M. D. (1990). Medical complications of intravenous drug use. *Journal of General Internal Medicine, 5,* 249–257.

Strain, E. C., Bigelow, G. E., Liebson, I. A., & Stitzer, M. L. (1999). Moderate- vs high-dose methadone in the treatment of opioid dependence: A randomized trial. *Journal of the American Medical Association, 281,* 1000–1005.

Strain, E. C., Stitzer, M. L., Liebson, I. A., & Bigelow, G. E. (1993). Dose-response effects of methadone in the treatment of opioid dependence. *Annals of Internal Medicine, 119,* 23–27.

Strain, E. C., Stitzer, M. L., Liebson, I. A., & Bigelow, G. E. (1994). Buprenorphine versus methadone in the treatment of opioid-dependent cocaine users. *Psychopharmacology (Berl), 116,* 401–406.

Strang, J., Bearn, J., & Gossop, M. (1997). Opiate detoxification under anaesthesia. *BMJ, 315,* 1249–1250.

Tennant, F. S., Jr., Russell, B. A., Casas, S. K., & Bleich, R. N. (1975). Heroin detoxification. A comparison of propoxyphene and methadone. *Journal of the American Medical Association, 232,* 1019–1022.

Tracqui, A., Kintz, P., & Ludes, B. (1998). Buprenorphine-related deaths among drug addicts in France: A report on 20 fatalities. *Journal of Analytical Toxicology, 22,* 430–434.

U.S. Preventive Services Task Force. (1996). *Guide to clinical preventive services* (2nd ed.). Baltimore: Williams & Wilkins.

Walsh, S. L., Preston, K. L., Stitzer, M. L., Cone, E. J., & Bigelow, G. E. (1994). Clinical pharmacology of buprenorphine: Ceiling effects at high doses. *Clinical Pharmacology and Therapeutics, 55,* 569–580.

Ward, J., Mattick, R. P., & Hall, W. (1998). The use of urinalysis during opioid replacement therapy. In J. Ward, R. P. Mattick, & W. Hall (Eds.), *Methadone maintenance treatment and other opioid replacement therapies* (p. 571). Amsterdam: Harwood.

Warner, E. A., Kosten, T. R., & O'Connor, P. G. (1997). Pharmacotherapy for opioid and cocaine abuse. *Medical Clinics of North America, 81,* 909–925.

Wyshak, G., & Modest, G. A. (1996). Violence, mental health, and substance abuse in patients who are seen in primary care settings. *Archives of Family Medicine, 5,* 441–447.

Yancovitz, S. R., Des Jarials, D. C., Peyser, N. P., Drew, E., Friedman, P., Trigg, H. L., et al. (1991). A randomized trial of an interim methadone maintenance clinic. *American Journal of Public Health, 81,* 1185–1191.

Ziedonis, D., & Brady, K. (1997). Dual diagnosis in primary care. Detecting and treating both the addiction and mental illness. *Medical Clinics of North America, 81,* 1017–1036.

Zielbauer, P. (1999, October 31). State knew of risky heroin treatment before patient deaths. *The New York Times,* p. 41.

Zweben, J. E., & Payte, J. T. (1990). Methadone maintenance in the treatment of opioid dependence. A current perspective. *Western Journal of Medicine, 152,* 588–599.

Chapter 8

Methadone versus L-alpha-acetylmethadol (LAAM) in the Treatment of Opiate Addiction

A Meta-Analysis of the Randomized, Controlled Trials

Morton Glanz, M.D., M.S.
Sidney Klawansky, M.D., Ph.D.
William McAuliffe, Ph.D.
Thomas Chalmers, M.D.

Heroin addiction continues to be an important menace to health and safety in the United States despite a committed public effort to control it. According to a recent survey, at least 500,000 individuals in the United States are currently estimated to be dependent on heroin or other opioids. This same survey suggested that about 1% of adults have tried heroin at least once (Gfroerer, 1996). Although generally perceived to be a drug of the 1960s, heroin is resurfacing as an important public health menace. Its use is rising, especially among young adult, middle income, and suburban groups. High purity and low cost are partially responsible for this escalation in popularity. Formerly addicted individuals are also being drawn back into drug use as a result of these factors (Office of National Drug Control Policy, 1996).

Despite the national interest in this problem, the treatment of heroin addiction remains generally problematic. To this point in time, there remain few good outcome studies on the differential treatment of this disorder. The reported success for these programs has varied widely (Ball et al., 1988; Hubbard et al., 1989; Stimmel et al., 1977). Success is usually measured by program-retention rate, illicit drug use, discontinuation of treatment because of side effects, or various measures of social functioning. Methadone maintenance programs remain a cornerstone of therapy for heroin addiction. A recent survey estimates that 115,000 patients are under treatment with methadone in 750 programs throughout the 42 states that offer such services (Institute of Medicine, 1995). Several randomized, controlled trials have documented the superiority of methadone over placebo in heroin addiction (Farrell et al., 1994). Nevertheless, the use of methadone in an addiction program involves certain inherent operational difficulties. Methadone has to be administered on a daily, resource-intensive fashion or with attendant take-home privileges with the associated risk of street diversion. Also, the stigma of the methadone clinic itself may deter addicted persons from seeking help.

L-alpha-acetylmethadol (LAAM), as an alternative to methadone, was introduced in the 1970s in response to these concerns. A synthetic analog of methadone, its 72- to 96-hour half-life theoretically allows for an every-third-day dosage schedule, thus freeing up both staff and patients for other aspects of the rehabilitation process. Also, the less demanding dosage scheduling has logistic advantages for treatment planning in sparsely populated regions, with the greater dispersion of rehabilitation candidates. Similarly, there are operational advantages for the medical-maintenance patient: the chronic stable patient is managed outside of a structured program (i.e., from the individual practioner's office) in an effort to separate him from the elements of the drug culture. Finally, LAAM may be less stigmatizing than methadone, not having the negative perception of methadone by segments of the street-addict population. Thus it could draw some clients into treatment who had avoided methadone (Ling, Rawson, & Compton, 1994).

Phase III trials were completed in the 1970s. These uniformly demonstrated safety equivalent to methadone and uneven, but generally favorable, levels of efficacy (Ling et al., 1976; Ling, Klett, & Roderic, 1978; Senay, Dorus, & Renault, 1977). There was a very long delay in the approval process in the United States. The FDA finally approved LAAM in 1993, despite the fact that it already had been intensely studied in over 4,000 patients over the previous 2 decades (Ling et al., 1994). For unclear reasons, the widespread subsequent adoption of LAAM in the treatment of heroin addiction has not ensued, despite the obvious operational advantages. By the end of 1994, only approximately 200 patients were receiving LAAM. Cited reasons include delays at the state regulatory and FDA/DEA licensing levels and disinterest by both program staff and patients (Prendergast et al., 1995). Currently, it is certainly possible that because all of the randomized trials are old, with results not definitively pointing to a treatment advantage for LAAM, there has been no incentive for planners to incorporate LAAM into their respective programs. However, a positive quantitative assessment of the relative efficacy of LAAM versus methadone regarding major endpoint measures might alter such perceptions, especially considering the operational advantages of LAAM as cited.

In this chapter, we undertake a meta-analysis of the reported randomized controlled trials in an effort to assess the relative overall efficacy of LAAM therapy as compared with methadone in heroin addiction. Previous overviews of LAAM therapy have not used quantitative methods to assess its efficacy (Ling et al., 1994; Prendergast et al., 1995; Tennant et al., 1985). Meta-analysis is a discipline that uses statistical methods to pool the data of reported trials and presents an objective, quantitative estimate of the efficacy of an intervention. In addition to producing a quantitative expression of the reported experience (as opposed to the traditional "review article" format) its strength lies in its ability to reduce the Type II error of individual smaller studies and thereby increase the level of certitude for or against a given treatment. A Type II error occurs in a study when a true outcome difference exists in the populations under study, however because of insufficient numbers of subjects studied, the consequently widened confidence intervals (CIs) do not allow for statistical significance to be inferred at the designated P level; that is, the null hypothesis is not rejected.

METHODS

A thorough literature search was conducted for randomized, controlled trials comparing methadone with LAAM therapy in the management of heroin addiction. This included a MEDLINE search (keywords: heroin addiction, methadone, levo-alpha-acetylmethadol) as well as a review of bibliographies of retrieved articles and pertinent review articles. The search spanned 1966 to 1996. Retrieved articles were evaluated for suitability of inclusion in a meta-analysis, looking for similar endpoints represented in at least three studies, because statistical considerations limit the pooling of fewer studies (Fleiss, 1993). The endpoints ultimately considered were illicit drug use, retention in treatment program, and discontinuance of treatment because of side effects (also designated as compliance).

The data extraction process often involves arbitrary decisions regarding the value chosen for an outcome variable. These situations were generally analyzed in a "conservative" manner, that is, that the new (LAAM) treatment was less efficacious. The data were analyzed using the Meta-Analyst software program for dichotomous variables (Joseph Lau, M.D., Boston, 1993). This program conducts a meta-analysis using both the Fixed Effects and Random Effects (DerSimonian-Laird) models. The former model considers all studies as samples emanating from a single universe of studies, and thus only utilizes the variances of the individual studies in computing a confidence interval for the pooled result of the analysis. The latter model assumes multiple universes of studies (manifested by a significant test result for "heterogeneity"), and thus considers both the variance of the individual studies and an overall variance for the sample of studies in computing the pooled confidence interval. This method is therefore more conservative; that is, a wider range of confidence is generated for a given data set. The results for each data set are reported in the form of a risk difference, odds ratio, and risk ratio, with a test of heterogeneity for each pooled statistic. The degree of heterogeneity is expressed as the Q statistic. By convention, when Q is greater than k-1, where k is the number of included studies, then heterogeneity is considered significant (Fleiss, 1993). We chose to use the risk difference to express the difference in outcome between the two treatment groups because of its advantages as cited by Mostellar and Laird (1990). These include the more facile applicability to the clinical situation and its normal sampling distribution even when there are small sample sizes.

Formal quality scoring was performed on these studies according to the method of Chalmers (1981). This exercise involves the assessment of critical aspects of a well-designed and well-executed controlled clinical trial, especially the randomization and blinding processes. A high "quality score" is dependent on rigorous documentation of these latter facets. The importance of descriptive and analytic data display and analysis is also stressed. The quality score is derived for potential use as a discriminating variable for inclusion, weighting, or sensitivity analysis regarding individual studies in the analysis.

RESULTS

The salient features of the included studies are displayed in Table 8.1. The data extracted for each endpoint are displayed in Table 8.2. The literature search identified a total of 14 randomized, controlled trials comparing methadone with LAAM in the treatment of heroin addiction (Crowley et al., 1985; Freedman & Czertko, 1981; Jaffe et al., 1970, 1972; Jaffe & Senay, 1971; Karp-Gelernter, Savage, & McCabe, 1982; Ling et al., 1976, 1978; Marcovici et al., 1981; Panell, Charuvastra, & Ouren, 1977; Savage et al., 1976; Senay et al., 1977; Sorensen, Hargreaves, & Weinberg, 1982; Zaks, Fink, & Freedman, 1972). The study dates ranged from 1970 to 1982. The number of subjects ranged from 10 to 636, with a median of 54. The study durations ranged from 3 to 52 weeks, with a median of 26. The combinable endpoints of program retention, illicit drug use, and compliance were identified in 11, 10, and 4 studies, respectively. The studies varied in design regarding some potentially important moderator variables. These included an open versus closed design, presence or absence of a stabilization/run-in period on methadone for both treatment arms, the option of dosage variability, and differences in dosing schedule.

Program retention was analyzed as an "all-or-none" phenomenon; that is, the patient had to remain in the program for the duration of the study to be considered as "retained." Although other researchers in the field have used the

TABLE 8.1. Study Characteristics

Study	n	Duration weeks	Blinding	Methadone Stabilization	LAAM Dosage	Dosing Structure	Urine Testing
Jaffe & Senay (1971)	10	3	Double-blind	Yes	N/A; meth./LAAM ratio: 1/1.2	Weekend, take-home, variable LAAM	Weekly
Jaffe et al. (1972)	34	15	Double-blind	No	36–80 mg	Daily dosage for both groups; variable LAAM	3 times/week
Zaks et al. (1972)	20	26	Open	Detox before study	30–50 mg, Group 1; 80 mg, Group 2	LAAM dosage 3 times/ week; variable LAAM	3 times/week
Ling et al. (1976)	330	40	Double-blind	No	30–80 mg	Daily dosage for both groups; fixed LAAM	Weekly
Savage et al. (1976)	99	26	Double-blind	No	N/A; meth./LAAM ratio: 1/1.3	Daily dosage for both groups; variable LAAM	1–3 times/week
Panell et al. (1977)	60	40	Double-blind	No	80 mg	Daily dosage for both groups; fixed LAAM	Weekly
Senay et al. (1977)	33	14	Open	Yes	33.3–39.8 mg	LAAM dose 3 times/week; variable LAAM	Weekly
Ling et al. (1978)	636	40	Open	Yes	60–69 mg, mean range	LAAM dose 3 times/week; variable LAAM	Weekly
Freedman & Czertko (1981)	48	52	Single-blind (to dose only)	Yes	mean 13.9 mg; meth./LAAM ratio: 1/1.3	LAAM dose 3 times/week; variable LAAM	2 times/week
Marcovici et al. (1981)	54	32	Open	No	46 mg average Mon. Wed.; 56 mg average Fri.	LAAM dose 3 times/week; variable LAAM	Not specified
Sorensen et al. (1982)	33	12	Double-blind	Detox only	30–40 mg	LAAM dose 3 timse/week; meth. supplement	2 times/week
Karp-Gelernter et al. (1982)	95	40	Double-blind	Yes	N/A; meth./LAAM ratio: 1/1	3- or 7-day schedule for meth. and LAAM; variable LAAM	1–3 times/week

Note: LAAM = L-alpha-acetylmethadol.

TABLE 8.2. Extracted Data for Outcome Variables

Study	n	Illicit drug use	Treatment retention	Discontinuation due to side effects
Jaffe & Senay (1971)	Meth.: 5	2/5		
	LAAM: 5	2/5		
Jaffe et al. (1972)	Meth.: 15	4/15	13/15	
	LAAM:19	10/19	14/19	
Zaks et al. (1972)	Meth.: 10	0/10	8/10	
	LAAM: 10	1/9	8/9	
Ling et al. (1976)	Meth. (50 mg): 146		74/142	4/142
	Meth. (100 mg): 142		44/142	10/142
	LAAM (80 mg): 142			
Savage et al. (1976)	Meth.: 52	3/52	31/52	14/52
	LAAM: 47	4/47	16/47	18/47
Panell et al. (1977)	Meth. (50 mg): 20		17/20	
	Meth. (100 mg): 20		12/20	
	LAAM: 20			
Senay et al. (1977)	Meth.: 96	27/96	72/96	
	LAAM: 97	25/97	51/97	
Ling et al. (1978)	Meth.: 308	166/306	184/306	0.306
	LAAM: 328	148/328	128/308	11/328
Freedman & Czertko	Meth.: 24	11/24	1/24	
(1981)	LAAM: 24	7/24	4/24	
Marcovici et al. (1981)	Meth.: 52	4/23	23/52	
	LAAM: 78	3/24	24/78	
Sorensen et al. (1982)	Meth.: 18	14/18	6/18	
	LAAM: 15	12/15	10/15	
Karp-Gelernter et al.	Meth.: 46	22/46	22/49	13/46
(1982)	LAAM: 49	27/49	17/49	18/49

Note: LAAM = L-alpha-acetylmethadol; Meth. = methadone.

actual number of days retained as an outcome variable, we were unable to do this and still pool all of the studies because of missing data in individual studies. For the illicit drug use data, individual studies reported either on individuals as positive with a positive urine at any point in time during the study, or the percentage of positive urines for the cohort as a whole. In the latter instance, the percentage was converted into a proportion by multiplying it by the number of individuals in the cohort. This product became the numerator of the derived proportion, with the number in the cohort used as the denominator. This transformation was required for the meta-analytic pooling process. Two excluded studies lacked data for these endpoints (Crowley et al., 1985; Jaffe et al., 1970). The Crowley et al. study measured mood and motility, endpoints not cited in any other study. The excluded Jaffe et al. (1970) study compared only symptoms between the two treatment groups. Although this type of information was also included in many of the other studies, it was generally not presented in a manner that was easily or meaningfully extracted for pooling in a meta-analysis.

Several studies compared LAAM with different doses of methadone. In such instances only the results from the higher dose were initially included in the analysis, because the higher dose resulted in greater efficacy. Indeed, a recently published randomized, controlled trial of various doses of methadone in this disorder did confirm the superior efficacy of higher doses for various endpoints, including treatment retention and illicit drug use (Strain et al., 1993). The robustness of the conclusions was tested in sensitivity analyses utilizing the results of the lower methadone dosage in place of the higher one (Table 8.3).

For each endpoint, the risk difference is defined as the proportion of patients in the LAAM group positive for the endpoint, minus the proportion in the methadone group positive for the endpoint. Thus, for illicit drug use and discontinuance of treatment because of side effects, the risk difference would be negative if LAAM were favored. For retention in treatment, the risk difference would be positive if LAAM were favored.

Illicit Drug Use

All studies with illicit drug use as an endpoint used urine testing as a means for detecting illicit drug use. Pooling of the 10 studies using the endpoint of illicit drug use, with the Fixed Effects Model, disclosed a mean risk difference of –0.02 (95% CI: –0.07 to 0.02) in favor of LAAM. For the Random Effects Model, the results were –0.01 (95% CI: –0.07 to 0.04). The risk difference here is defined as the proportion of patients with any illicit drug use in the LAAM group, minus the proportion of illicit drug use in the methadone group. Thus, the negative sign denotes a lower mean usage in the LAAM treatment groups. However, this finding was not statistically significant ($P \leq 0.35$), given that the CI overlapped the null (0.00) value. The Q statistic for heterogeneity was 10.74, which was significant. Therefore, the random effects model was utilized.

Patient Retention in Treatment Program

Program retention was defined as the proportion of patients remaining in the assigned treatment arm of the study until its completion. The risk difference is defined as the proportion of patients retained in the LAAM group minus the proportion of patients retained in the methadone group. Pooling of the data, using the Fixed Effects Model, resulted in a mean risk difference in dropout rate of –0.17 (95% CI: –0.21 to –0.12) in favor of methadone. Using the Random Effects Model, the mean risk difference was –0.13 (95% CI: –0.21 to –0.04) in favor of methadone. Both results were significant ($P<0.003$), not

TABLE 8.3. Sensitivity Analysis

Endpoint	Karp-Gelernter et al. (1982) Initial	Karp-Gelernter et al. (1982) Adjusted	Ling et al. (1976) Initial	Ling et al. (1976) Adjusted	Panell et al. (1977) Initial	Panell et al. (1977) Adjusted	Initial Pooled Result	Adjusted Pooled Result
Compliance	Meth.: 13/46 LAAM: 18/49	Meth.: 8/22 LAAM: 9/27	Meth.: 4/142 LAAM: 10/142	Meth.: 5/288 LAAM: 10/142			0.4 (0.02 to 0.05) fixed effects	0.04 (0.02 to 0.05) fixed effects
Retention	Meth.: 22/49 LAAM: 17/49	Meth.: 8/22 LAAM: 8/27	Meth.: 74/142 LAAM: 44/142	Meth.: 135/288 LAAM: 44/142	Meth.: 17/20 LAAM: 12/20	Meth.: 31/40 LAAM: 12/20	−0.13 (−0.21 to −0.04) random effects	−0.11 (−0.19 to −0.03) random effects
Illicit drug use	Meth.: 22/46 LAAM: 27/49	Meth.: 1/22 LAAM: 14/27					−0.01 (−0.07 to 0.04) random effects	−0.02 (−0.08 to 0.03) random effects

Note: LAAM = L-alpha-acetylmethadol; Meth. = methadone.

overlapping the null (0.00) value. The Q statistic for heterogeneity was 27.20, which was statistically significant. Therefore, the random effects result was considered the more valid result.

Discontinuation of Treatment Because of Side Effects (Compliance)

This endpoint was defined as the proportion of the patients discontinuing a study treatment specifically because of side effects (but still remaining in the program itself). The risk difference was taken as the proportion of patients discontinuing treatment in the LAAM group, minus the proportion discontinuing treatment in the control group. Pooling this data with the Fixed Effects Model produced a statistically significant mean risk difference in treatment discontinuance of 0.04 (95% CI: 0.02 to 0.05; $P<0.0001$) in favor of methadone therapy. The Q statistic for heterogeneity was 1.34, which was not significant. Therefore, the fixed and random effects analyses produced the same result.

Sensitivity Analysis

As is often the case in conducting a meta-analysis, the data extraction process involved certain judgments on the part of the investigators. In three studies, two different data subsets were available for the methadone arms of the study. In two studies (Ling et al., 1976; Panell et al., 1977), this involved two different dosages (50 mg and 100 mg) of methadone. The higher dosage groups performed better, as expected, and were utilized in the initial pooling process. Similarly, the Karp-Galernter et al. (1982) study had groups who received methadone or LAAM, with 3- or 7-day-per-week mandatory clinic attendance schedules. The thrice-weekly groups fared better regarding the retention endpoint, again as expected. The values for the 3- and 7-day groups for each drug were combined in the initial meta-analysis. This, of course, does not reflect the actual schedules for either drug in practice. Only requiring clinic attendance three times a week (for methadone therapy) biases the analysis in favor of this treatment, as does requiring daily attendance for LAAM administration. Thus, the initial overall analysis should have been biased in favor of methadone.

For the sensitivity analysis, both dosage groups were included in the analysis in the case of the Ling et al. (1976) and Panell et al. (1977) studies. For the Karp-Galernter et al. study (1982), only the thrice-weekly attendance LAAM group was compared with the daily-attendance methadone group, thus mirroring the schedules that would actually occur in practice.

The changes in the data for the individual studies, the resultant changes in the pooled mean risk differences, and associated CIs and levels of significance are displayed in Table 8.3. For each study and associated endpoint involved in the sensitivity analysis, the table shows the initial and subsequently adjusted raw data. The final two columns show how the pooled result changes when the adjusted data are utilized in the overall analysis. As can be seen, in no instance were the conclusions of the original meta-analysis altered by the sensitivity analysis exercise.

Quality Scoring

The results of the formal quality scoring were as follows: Freedman and Czertko (1981): 0.36; Marcovici et al. (1981): 0.37; Zaks et al. (1972): 0.30; Jaffe and Senay (1971): 0.37; Senay et al. (1977): 0.39; Panell et al. (1977): 0.46; Ling et al. (1978): 0.51; Sorensen et al. (1982): 0.57; Karp-Galernter (1982): 0.58; Jaffe et al. (1972): 0.64; Ling et al. (1976): 0.69; Savage et al. (1976): 0.73. The scores are expressed as a ratio of total number of points over total possible points. The mean score was 0.50 ± 0.14. These scores are similar in magnitude to those noted in a survey of randomized controlled clinical trials (Reitman, Sacks, & Chalmers, 1987). All scores were within two standard deviations of the mean score. Given the absence of significant outliers, no trials were excluded from the analysis on the basis of the quality score.

DISCUSSION

The results of our meta-analysis of available randomized, controlled trials comparing LAAM to methadone in heroin addiction therapy show no difference in the level of illicit drug use and small but statistically significant benefits for methadone in patient retention and discontinuance-of-treatment-because-of-side-effects endpoints. These findings were fairly consistent regardless of the pooling model utilized or the choices made for the specified arbitrary aspects of the data extraction process, as explored in the sensitivity analysis.

   In a study of this nature it is important to assess the clinical significance of the findings as well as to explore any modifying factors that could have influenced the outcome. A very important consideration is the relative importance of the three different endpoints used in this study. Ling et al. (1994) are of the strong opinion that the urine test data, reflecting illicit drug use, provide the most meaningful criterion of program efficacy. Hubbard et al.'s (1989) comprehensive 1989 analysis of treatment outcome for over 10,000 substance abusers, however, suggests that treatment retention may be the endpoint of overriding importance.

   There are reasons to consider that the higher retention rate in the methadone groups was not entirely due to the differential pharmacological properties of the agents involved. Both staff and patients were well aware of the "experimental" nature of LAAM therapy. Given the already inherently suspicious nature of the addict subculture, it would not be surprising to find a lack of trust or tolerance for the "new" treatment. The fact that some of the trials were closed does not mitigate against this concern, as it seems clear that because of the different pharmacokinetics of the two agents, patients could distinguish between the two drugs. Specifically, because of a much more rapid rise to peak blood level (of active metabolite), methadone tends to be much more euphoriogenic. In many of the trials, the LAAM patient was able to return to methadone treatment should he or she no longer wish to continue in the study (i.e., to take LAAM). The methadone subjects, of course, could only return to street sources of supply. Indeed, the open Ling et al. study saw much higher rates of transfer from LAAM to methadone than did the closed trial. Thus there was an inherent a priori structural bias against LAAM.

Besides blinding, the program-structural elements of variability of LAAM dosing, the presence of a methadone stabilization period before LAAM treatment, and the use of higher Friday LAAM dosage could affect the success of a program (Brown, Watters, & Inglemart, 1982/1983; Ling et al., 1976; Tennant et al., 1986). As noted in Table 8.1, these elements were variably present in the included studies.

The significance of the mean difference in retention rate of 13% (random effects model) for methadone treatment, ignoring potential confounding factors as outlined above, is, in itself, uncertain. The magnitude of this difference relative to the overall retention rates and cost–benefit factors as applied to the population at risk are of importance. Given the overall 58% weighted average retention rate for the methadone groups of the included studies, 13% would represent a moderate proportion of this overall rate. In a discussion of what constitutes "clinically meaningful results" in a generic sense, Sackett et al. (1991) noted that the finding of a 25% difference between treatments will induce many to choose that particular treatment, whereas a difference of 50% will cause most clinicians to do so. These investigators also use a computation designated as "number needed to treat," or NNT. This is the inverse of the risk difference and defines how many subjects must be treated with the preferred therapy for a single subject to actually benefit from it. In this instance, 1/0.13, or 8, would have to be given methadone over LAAM to prevent one subject from dropping out. Although quite arbitrary, this value is considered to represent a relatively lower range of efficacy (Moreland & Thomson, 1994). On the other hand, this risk difference in a macroeconomic, cost-benefit sense, could well prove to be quite important. Hubbard's data do indeed suggest that this difference is important in the latter sense. This study shows the various indices of treatment closely linked to program retention and the benefits of methadone maintenance as quantified in economic terms to be highly leveraged. Thus the statistically significant difference in retention noted in our study, even in just looking at the lower end of the CIs, would suggest concluding this analysis in favor of methadone.

This analysis regarding the importance and validity of the retention endpoint would also be relevant in considering the importance of the small but statistically significant difference in treatment-discontinuation-because-of-side-effects endpoint in favor of methadone.

Thus, retention and treatment discontinuation differences notwithstanding, if the thrice-weekly dosage schedule of LAAM treatment, as opposed to the daily regimen of the methadone program, would free up resources to improve access to the programs or free up counseling resources within a program, then these benefits particular to the less-frequent dosing schedule and the attraction of clients who would not use methadone could at least partially offset the putatively lower rate of retention and higher loss due to side effects.

The Tennant et al. (1986) report on LAAM therapy does indeed support the idea that it may, in fact, be preferable to methadone for select groups of patients. In that study, 39% reported that if LAAM were not available they would return to heroin or attempt drug abstinence before they would reenter methadone treatment.

A discussion of these results would be incomplete without touching on the role in general of meta-analysis in clinical medicine. Just how third-party payers, policy analysts, and practicing clinicians should respond to the conclusions of a meta-analysis was the subject of a recent review (Borzak & Ridker, 1995). It is argued that a meta-analysis cannot be ascribed the hypothesis-testing validity of a large, prospective, randomized controlled trial. By nature, it is reduced to a more descriptive or hypothesis-generating function. Although this purist view may be true in theory, for many clinical problems, the large prospective trials necessary to reach a "valid" conclusion may never be forthcoming. As the authors of the review conclude, in assessing the imperfect state of knowledge for many situations, the clinician must resort to "a considered review of the totality of evidence from pathophysiologic principles, to basic laboratory research, meta-analyses, and individual trials" (Borzak & Ridker, 1995).

CONCLUSIONS

A meta-analysis of the reported randomized controlled trials of LAAM versus methadone therapy for heroin addiction shows a statistically significant advantage for methadone in what may well be the most important endpoint: treatment retention. The endpoint of illicit drug use showed no significant difference but did produce a trend in favor of LAAM. Treatment discontinuance did show a small but statistically significant difference in favor of methadone. There are several important potential causes for these findings above and beyond the intrinsic characteristics of the two drugs themselves. Even if valid, the clinical and fiscal importance of these differences are uncertain. Given the potential practical and operational benefits of LAAM therapy over methadone in certain situations, it would seem reasonable at this point to support and encourage LAAM therapy as an important alternative to methadone.

REFERENCES

Ball, J. C., Lange, W. R., Myers, C. P., et al. (1988). Reducing the risk of AIDS through methadone maintenance. *Journal of Health and Social Behavior, 29,* 214–226.

Borzak, S., & Ridker, P. M. (1995). Discordance between meta-analyses and large-scale randomized, controlled trials. *Annals of Internal Medicine, 123,* 873–877.

Brown, B. S., Watters, J. K., & Inglemart, A. S. (1982/1983). Methadone maitainence dosage levels and program retention. *American Journal of Drug and Alcohol Abuse, 9,* 129–139.

Chalmers, T. C. (1981). A method for assessing the quality of randomized controlled trials. *Controlled Clinical Trials, 2,* 31–49.

Crowley, T. J., Macdonald, M. J., Wagner, J. E., et al. (1985). Acetylmethadol vs methadone: Human mood and motility. *Psychopharmacology, 86,* 458–463.

Farrell, M., Ward, J., Mattick, R., et al. (1994). Methadone maintenance treatment in opiate dependence: A review. *BMJ, 304,* 997–1001.

Fleiss, J. L. (1993). The statistical basis of meta-analysis. *Statistical Methods in Medical Research, 2,* 121–145.

Freedman, R. R., & Czertko, G. (1981). A comparison of thrice-weekly LAAM and daily methadone in employed heroin addicts. *Drug and Alcohol Dependence, 8,* 215–222.

Gfroerer, J. C. (1996). Office of Applied Studies, SAMHSA. *Preliminary estimates from the 1995 National Household Survey on Drug Abuse.* Advance Report Number 18. Rockville, MD: SAMHSA, Office of Applied Studies.

Hubbard, R. L., Marsden, M. E., Rachel, J. V., et al. (1989). *Drug abuse treatment: A national study of effectiveness.* Chapel Hill, NC: University of North Carolina Press.

Institute of Medicine. (1995). *Federal regulation of methadone treatment.* Washington, DC: National Academy Press.

Jaffe, J. H., Schuster, C. H., Smith, B., et al. (1970). Comparison of acetylmethadol and methadone in the treatment of long-term heroin users: A pilot study. *Journal of the American Medical Association, 211,* 1834–1836.

Jaffe, J. H., & Senay, E. C. (1971). Methadone and L-methadyl acetate use in management of narcotics addicts. *Journal of the American Medical Association, 216,* 1303–1305.

Jaffe, J. A., Senay, E. C., Schuster, C. R., et al. (1972). Methadyl acetate vs methadone: A double-blind study in heroin users. *Journal of the American Medical Association, 222,* 437–442.

Karp-Gelernter, E., Savage, C., & McCabe, O. L. (1982). Evaluation of clinic schedules for LAAM and methadone: A controlled study. *International Journal of Addiction, 17,* 805–813.

Ling, W., Charuvastra, C., Kaim, S. C., et al. (1976). Methadyl acetate and methadone as maintenance treatments for heroin addicts. *Archives of General Psychiatry, 33,* 709–719.

Ling, W., Klett, J., & Roderic, D. G. (1978). A cooperative clinical study of methadyl acetate. *Archives of General Psychiatry, 35,* 345–353.

Ling, W., Rawson, R. A., & Compton, M. A. (1994, April–June). Substitution pharmacotherapies for opioid addiction: From methadone to LAAM and buprenorphine. *Journal of Psychoactive Drugs, 26,* 119–128.

Marcovici, M., O'Brien, C., McLellan, A. T., et al. (1981). A clinical controlled study of L-alpha-acetylmethadol in the treatment of narcotic addiction. *American Journal of Psychiatry, 138,* 234–236.

Moreland, J., & Thomson, M. A. (1994). Efficacy of electromyographic biofeedback compared to conventional physical therapy for upper extremity function following stroke: A research overview and meta-analysis. *Physical Therapy, 74,* 534–547.

Mostellar, F., & Laird, N. (1990). Some statistical methods for combining results. *International Journal of Technology Assessment in Health Care, 6,* 5–30.

Office of National Drug Control Policy. (1996, Spring). *Pulse check: National trends in drug abuse.* Washington, DC: Executive Office of the President.

Panell, J., Charuvastra, V. C., & Ouren, J. (1977). Methadyl acetate vs. methadone: The experience of one hospital. *Medical Journal of Australia, 2,* 150–152.

Prendergast, M. L., Grella, C., Perry, S. M., et al. (1995). Levo-alpha-acetyl-methadol (LAAM): Clinical, research, and policy issues of a new pharmacotherapy for opioid addiction. *Journal of Psychoactive Drugs, 27,* 239–246.

Reitman, D., Sacks, H. S., & Chalmers, T. C. (1987). Technical quality assessment of randomized controlled trials (abstract). *Controlled Clinical Trials, 8,* 282.

Sackett, D., Haynes, R. B., Guyatt, G., et al. (1991). *Clinical epidemiology: A basic science* (2nd ed.). Boston: Little, Brown.

Savage, C., Karp, E. G., Curran, S. F., et al. (1976). Methadone/LAAM maintenance: A comparison study. *Comprehensive Psychiatry, 17,* 415–424.

Senay, E. C., Dorus, W., & Renault, P. F. (1978). Methadyl acetate and methadone: An open comparison. *Journal of the American Medical Association, 237,* 138–142.

Sorensen, J. L., Hargreaves, W. A., & Weinberg, J. A. (1982). Withdrawal from heroin in three or six weeks. *Archives of General Psychiatry, 39,* 167–171.

Stimmel, B., Goldberg, J., Rotkopf, E., et al. (1977). Ability to remain abstinent after methadone detoxification: A six-year study. *Journal of the American Medical Association, 237,* 1216–1220.

Strain, E. C., Stitzer, M. L., Liebson, I. A., et al. (1993). Dose-response effects of methadone in the treatment of opioid dependence. *Annals of Internal Medicine, 199,* 23–27.

Tennant, F. S., Rawson, R. A., Pumprey, E., et al. (1986). Clinical experiences with 959 opioid-dependent patients treated with L-alpha acetylmethadol (LAAM). *Journal of Substance Abuse Treatment, 3,* 195–202.

Zaks, A., Fink, M., & Freedman, A. M. (1972). Levomethadyl in maintenance treatment of opiate dependence. *Journal of the American Medical Association, 220,* 811–813.

Chapter 9

Old Psychotherapies for Cocaine Dependence Revisited

Kathleen M. Carroll, Ph.D.

The publication of the results of the National Institute on Drug Abuse Collaborative Cocaine Treatment Study (CCTS; Crits-Christoph et al., 1999) like the publication of and comments on some of the first pharmacologic trials in *Archives of General Psychiatry* a decade ago (Arndt, Dorozynsky, Woody, McLellan, & O'Brien, 1992; Kosten, Morgan, Falcioni, & Schottenfeld, 1992; Meyer, 1992), denotes a landmark in the development and evaluation of treatments for cocaine dependence. Since 1992, myriad pharmacotherapies have failed to demonstrate efficacy against the Goliath of cocaine dependence. Instead, "weak" approaches, such as psychotherapy, have emerged as the David of this field; note that the review by Meyer in 1992 of the state of pharmacotherapies for cocaine dependence ended with the words "lest we forget the importance and efficacy of nonpharmacological treatments." Behavioral therapies, in particular contingency management approaches (Higgins et al., 1991, 1994; Higgins, Budney, Bickel, & Hughes, 1993; Silverman et al., 1996, 1998), have been demonstrated to be effective and sufficient treatments for most cocaine-dependent patients who receive them. While important efforts continue to identify effective pharmacotherapies, the results of this excellent study (CCTS) highlight several points deserving further comment, including (a) poor retention but generally good improvement across treatments; (b) failure to replicate an earlier study on the effects of professional psychotherapy versus disease-model approaches for methadone-maintained opiate addicts; and (c) the need to distinguish the therapies evaluated in the CCTS from other behavioral treatments demonstrated to be effective for cocaine dependence. First, however, this outstanding group of investigators is to be applauded on an extraordinarily well-conducted study, and in particular on their use of the most rigorous methods to define and implement the treatments studied, which make these findings so compelling.

LESS IS OFTEN MORE

Ever since cocaine abusers began seeking treatment, researchers and clinicians have noted how difficult it is to retain them in treatment, so much so that retention has become more or less a proxy for treatment "success." The CCTS, which offered intensive psychotherapy (36 individual and 24 group sessions for 24 weeks—a total of 60 sessions), had poor retention, with patients on average completing less than half of sessions offered, and only 28% completing treatment.

However, it is difficult to compare retention in this study with other outpatient studies of cocaine abusers because of the practice used here of selecting for individuals who completed a 2-week orientation phase prior to randomization, which resulted in loss of almost half of the eligible study population (383 of 870), and apparently individuals with more severe cocaine use and other problems (Sisqueland et al., 1998). The orientation procedure might be seen as an effective intervention in itself, as the figures suggest the bulk of the reduction in cocaine use occurred during this early period, with comparatively fewer reductions for the remainder of treatment. Thus, it is possible to interpret the study as evaluating the effects of intensive psychotherapy on a lower severity sample who were motivated to seek additional psychotherapy after having already made substantial reductions in their cocaine use. Thus, the poor retention does not suggest that the treatments offered were ineffective; instead, it is likely that too much treatment was offered to this select sample, and briefer versions of these treatments may have been sufficient.

Another issue with impractical expectations regarding any protocol's ability to retain participants is subsequent methodological problems. For example, it was not possible to use biological measures such as urine toxicology screens as an outcome measure, as only 43% of the weekly urine samples were collected, leading to reliance on self-report data. Compliance bias is another potential problem, as rates of follow-up at 3 and 6 months after treatment seemed somewhat higher for the better retained groups (cognitive therapy [CT] and supportive-expressive [SE] therapy) than the drug counseling groups.

TREATMENTS AND MODELS OF TREATMENT EVALUATION MAY NOT BE INTERCHANGEABLE ACROSS DRUG TYPES

The CCTS adapted all of its treatments and much of its basic design from those used in another landmark study of psychotherapy for opioid dependence, where SE and CT were contrasted with drug counseling among methadone-maintained opioid addicts (Woody et al., 1983; 1987). Thus, SE and CT had strong prior empirical support as treatment for stabilized opioid addicts; however, no data existed on the efficacy of these approaches with cocaine-dependent populations when this study began.

In the studies by Woody et al. (1983, 1987), the two professional psychotherapies were essentially evaluated as "add-ons" to methadone maintenance and contrasted with drug counseling alone. Both SE and CT were found to enhance outcome, particularly for patients with higher psychiatric severity and those with antisocial personality disorder. Essentially the same study, with similar hypotheses regarding main and matching effects, was conducted here, with group drug counseling essentially substituting for methadone maintenance as in the studies by Woody et al. (although with a more restricted range of psychiatric severity in the CCTS). The results of the two studies are quite different, pointing to limitations of assuming interchangeability of models of treatment and study design for opioid- versus cocaine-dependent subjects.

TREATMENTS FOR DRUG ABUSE
SHOULD TARGET DRUG ABUSE FIRST

A major finding from the CCTS is the comparatively good outcomes seen with the individual drug counseling condition, a manualized approach that draws heavily from 12-step philosophy. This finding, while striking, is not exactly surprising after several major recent studies have indicated that manualized, disease-model treatments are as effective and durable as other treatments with stronger levels of prior empirical support, including Project MATCH (1997) and a study of alcoholic cocaine abusers by our group (Carroll, Nich, Ball, McCance, & Rounsaville, 1998). This should not be interpreted as meaning that merely sending patients to self-help meetings constitutes sufficient treatment, however, as that is unlikely to be the case. Instead, manualized individual approaches drawn from widely used disease-model approaches and delivered by carefully selected and trained therapists can be as effective as professional psychotherapies for many cocaine abusers. The possible mechanisms for this—focus on abstinence and facilitating enduring relationships with supportive networks of other abstinent individuals—should be the subject of future investigations.

Another possible interpretation of these findings is that it may not be wise to change theoretical horses in midstream: the stabilization period that preceded randomization involved at least 3 sessions that encouraged attendance at self-help meetings and resulted in many patients having been exposed to 12-step principles prior to receiving SE or CT (Weiss et al., 1996). Possible "diluting" of SE and CT in this manner, combined with their primary emphases on substance-related problems that may have been less applicable to a more select sample (e.g., primary focus on interpersonal themes or cognitions related to drug abuse) may have reduced their effectiveness here.

Both SE and CT are also different in this manner from two approaches that have been demonstrated to be effective with many populations of cocaine abusers, contingency management (Higgins et al., 1991, 1993, 1994; Silverman et al., 1996, 1998) and cognitive-behavioral therapy (Carroll et al., 1998; Carroll, Rounsaville, Gordon, et al., 1994; Carroll, Rounsaville, Nich, et al., 1994; McKay et al., 1997; Maude-Griffin et al., 1998), both of which emphasize abstinence and strategies to achieve it. It is notable that in a recent study of alcoholic cocaine abusers by our group, cognitive-behavioral therapy was found to be as effective as a manualized 12-step facilitation approach, and significantly more effective than a supportive control condition (Carroll et al., 1998).

More generally, the CCTS illustrates a common problem for behavioral research in the addictions, namely, selection of appropriate "control" conditions against which to evaluate the effectiveness of new behavioral approaches. Until recently, many of us assumed, incorrectly, the inferiority of "treatment as usual" approaches that relied heavily on disease-model concepts. Our efforts to specify these approaches have resulted in our proving (to ourselves at least) just how effective they can be. When carefully conducted, as in the CCTS, they are not by any means a "placebo" treatment. It is the onus of treatment researchers to develop approaches that are more effective than, or at least as effective as, these. "Old" psychotherapies that relied on pharmacologic platforms like methadone to foster abstinence and address drug craving appear less applicable to cocaine dependence; "new" therapies must attend to old problems, particularly helping patients initiate and maintain abstinence.

REFERENCES

Arndt, I. O., Dorozynsky, L., Woody, G. E., McLellan, A. T., & O'Brien, C. P. (1992). Desipramine treatment of cocaine dependence in methadone-maintained patients. *Archives of General Psychiatry, 49,* 888–893.

Carroll, K. M., Nich, C., Ball, S. A., McCance, E., & Rounsaville, B. J. (1998). Treatment of cocaine and alcohol dependence with psychotherapy and disulfiram. *Addiction, 93,* 713–728.

Carroll, K. M., Rounsaville, B. J., Gordon, L. T., Nich, C., Jatlow, P., Bisighini, R. M., & Gawin, F. H. (1994). Psychotherapy and pharmacotherapy for ambulatory cocaine abusers. *Archives of General Psychiatry, 51,* 177–187.

Carroll, K. M., Rounsaville, B. J., Nich, C., Gordon, L. T., Wirtz, P. W., & Gawin, F. (1994). One-year follow-up of psychotherapy and pharmacotherapy for cocaine dependence. *Archives of General Psychiatry, 51,* 989–997.

Crits-Christoph, P., Siqueland, L., Blaine, J., Frank, A., Luborsky, L., Onken, L. S., Muenz, L. R., Thase, M. E., Weiss, R. D., Gastfriend, D. R., Woody, G. E., Barber, J. P., Butler, S. F., Daley, D., Salloum, I., Bishop, S., Najavits, L. M., Lis, J., Mercer, D., Griffin, M. L., Moras, K., & Beck, A. T. (1999). Psychosocial treatments for cocaine dependence: National Institute on Drug Abuse Collaborative Cocaine Study. *Archives of General Psychiatry, 56,* 493–502.

Higgins, S. T., Budney, A. J., Bickel, W. K., Foerg, F. E., Donham, R., & Badger, G. J. (1994). Incentives improve outcome in outpatient behavioral treatment of cocaine dependence. *Archives of General Psychiatry, 51,* 568–576.

Higgins, S. T., Budney, A. J., Bickel, W. K., & Hughes, J. R. (1993). Achieving cocaine abstinence with a behavioral approach. *American Journal of Psychiatry, 150,* 763–769.

Higgins, S. T., Delaney, D. D., Budney, A. J., Bickel, W. K., Hughes, J. R., Foerg, F., & Fenwick, J. W. (1991). A behavioral approach to achieving initial cocaine abstinence. *American Journal of Psychiatry, 148,* 1218–1224.

Kosten, T. R., Morgan, C. M., Falcioni, J., & Schottenfeld, R. S. (1992). Pharmacotherapy for cocaine-abusing methadone-maintained patients using amantidine or desipramine. *Archives of General Psychiatry, 49,* 894–898.

Maude-Griffin, P. M., Hohenstein, J. I. M., Humfleet, G. L., Reilley, P. M., Tusel, D. J., & Hall, S. M. (1998). Superior efficacy of cognitive-behavioral therapy for crack cocaine abusers. *Journal of Consulting and Clinical Psychology, 66,* 832–837.

McKay, J. R., Alterman, A. I., Cacciola, J. S., Rutherford, M. J., O'Brien, C. P., & Koppenhaver, J. (1997). Group counseling versus individualized relapse prevention aftercare following intensive outpatient treatment for cocaine dependence. *Journal of Consulting and Clinical Psychology, 65,* 778–788.

Meyer, R. E. (1992). New pharmacotherapies for cocaine dependence . . . revisited. *Archives of General Psychiatry, 49,* 900–904.

Project MATCH Research Group. (1997). Matching alcohol treatments to client heterogeneity: Project MATCH posttreatment drinking outcomes. *Journal of Studies on Alcohol, 58,* 7–29.

Silverman, K., Higgins, S. T., Brooner, R. K., Montoya, I. D., Cone, E. J., Schuster, C. R., & Preston, K. L. (1996). Sustained cocaine abstinence in methadone maintenance patients through voucher-based reinforcement therapy. *Archives of General Psychiatry, 53,* 409–415.

Silverman, K., Wong, C. J., Umbricht-Schneiter, A., Montoya, J. D., Schuster, C. R., & Preston, K. L. (1998). Broad beneficial effects of cocaine abstinence reinforcement among methadone patients. *Journal of Consulting and Clinical Psychology, 66,* 811–824.

Siqueland, L., Crits-Christoph, P., Frank, A., Daley, D., Weiss, R., Chittams, J., Blaine, J., & Luborsky, L. (1998). Predictors of dropout from psychosocial treatment of cocaine dependence. *Drug and Alcohol Dependence, 52,* 1–13.

Weiss, R. D., Griffin, M. L., Najavits, L. M., Hufford, C., Kogan, J., Thompson, H. J., Albeck, J. H., Bishop, S., Daley, D. C., Mercer, D., & Siqueland, L. (1996). Self-help activities in cocaine-dependent patients entering treatment. *Drug and Alcohol Dependence, 43,* 79–86.

Woody, G. E., Luborsky, L., McLellan, A. T., O'Brien, C. P., Beck, A. T., Blaine, J., Herman, I., & Hole, A. (1983). Psychotherapy for opiate addicts; does it help? *Archives of General Psychiatry, 40,* 639–645.

Woody, G. E., McLellan, A. T., Luborsky, L., & O'Brien, C. P. (1987). Twelve-month follow-up of psychotherapy for opiate dependence. *American Journal of Psychiatry, 144,* 590–596.

Chapter 10

New Treatments for Smoking Cessation

John R. Hughes, M.D.

MOTIVATING SMOKERS

Most clinician interactions with smokers involve motivating smokers to make a quit attempt. Protocols for such interactions using a brief intervention (2 to 5 minutes) have been well described in brochures from the National Cancer Institute (Glynn & Manley, 1989), the Agency for Health Care Policy Research (AHCPR; Smoking Cessation, 1996), and the American Psychiatric Association (Hughes et al., 1996; see Table 10.1). If a smoker does decide to quit, the clinician is faced with the dilemma of selecting a treatment. How does one decide which, if any, of the proven treatments to recommend? This chapter reviews the pros and cons of the several treatment options for smoking cessation and illustrates how these can be delivered within a brief intervention.

Writing of this article was supported by a Research Scientist Development Award DA-00109 from NIDA.

Dr. Hughes notes that in 1999, he received consulting fees, grants, and honoraria from Atlantic resources, BASF/Knoll, Capitol Associates, Elan/Sano, Glaxo Wellcome, INOVA Health Systems, Johnson, Bassin and Shaw, Mayo Medical Foundation, McNeil Pharmaceutical, MD Anderson Cancer Center, Medisphere, National Institutes of Health, Ness, Oregon Research Institute, Pharmacia & Upjohn, Pinney Associates, Prospect Associates, Pyramid Communications, Robert Wood Johnson Foundation, Sandler-Recht Communications, SmithKline Beecham Consumer Healthcare, Study Group on Analgesics and Nephropathy, University of Alabama at Birmingham, University of California at San Diego, University of Miami, Veterans Administration, Walker Law Firm, and World Health Organization.

TABLE 10.1. Contact Information for Smoking Cessation Resources or Referrals to Specialists

National Organizations

American Academy of Addiction Psychiatry
7301 Mission Road, Suite 252
Prairie Village, KS 66208
Phone: (913) 262-6161
www.aaap.org

American Cancer Society
1599 Clifton Road, NE
Atlanta, GA 30329-4251
Phone: (800) ACS-2345
www.cancer.org

American Lung Association
1740 Broadway
New York, NY 10019
Phone: (800) LUNG-USA
www.lungusa.org

American Psychiatric Association
1400 K Street NW
Washington, DC 20005
Phone: (202) 682-6239
www.apa.org

American Society of Addiction Medicine
4601 North Park Ave, Arcade
Suite 101
Chevy Chase, MD 20815
Phone: (301) 656-3920
www.asam.org

National Cancer Institute
9000 Rockville Pike
Building 31 10A16
Bethesday, MD 20892
Phone: (800) 4-CANCER
www.nci.nih.gov

Nicotine Anonymous
NAWSO
PO Box 591777
San Francisco, CA 94159-1777
Phone: (415) 750-0328
www.nicotine-anonymous.org

Society for Behavior Medicine
7611 Elmwood Avenue
Middletown, WI 53562
Phone: (800) LUNG-USA
Phone: (800) 827-7267
www.sbmweb.org

Society for Research on Nicotine & Tobacco
7611 Elmwood Avenue
Middleton, WI 53562
Phone: (608) 836-3787
www.srnt.org

Local Organizations

Your local hospital or worksite
    wellness/ Employee Assistance Program
Your state Department of Health
Your state alcohol and drug abuse office

Consumer Brochures

Treatment Works When You Choose to Stop Smoking
American Psychiatric Association
$19.95/12 (order #2525)
(202) 682-6268

Quit Smoking Action Plan
American Lung Association
(212) 315-8700
www.lungusa.org

Smart Move! A Stop Smoking Guide
American Cancer Society
(800) ACS-2345

Pharmaceutical Company Helplines

Glaxo Wellcome (bupropion)
800-822-6784 (UCAN-QUIT)
McNeil Consumer (OTC patch)
800-699-5765
Novartis Consumer (Rx patch)
800-452-0051
SmithKline Beecham (OTC patch)
800-834-5895
SmithKline Beecham (OTC gum)
800-419-4766

MOTIVATING YOURSELF, THE CLINICIAN

In this era of increasing financial and legal pressures, it is understandable that clinicians may find it difficult to remember to intervene with their patients who have a disorder that is asymptomatic, is not immediately life-threatening, could be self-cured, is unresponsive to treatment 80% of the time, and is often not considered their responsibility. On the other hand, clinicians' primary interest is promoting the health of their patients, and several studies have shown that the time spent on smoking cessation advice is *the* most effective use of a practitioner's time in terms of preventing mortality or morbidity (Cromwell et al., 1997). In fact, as smoking will cause the deaths of 50% of current smokers (U.S. Department of Health and Human Services, 1990) and as most smoking-related illnesses are reversible (Giovino et al., 1995), one premature death will have been avoided with every two smokers a clinician persuades and helps to stop smoking. Thus, a clinician who motivates 10 smokers to stop smoking in a year will have prevented five avoidable early deaths. Not a bad return on a total investment of a few hours.

SOME BASIC FACTS ABOUT SMOKING

About 30% of patients are current smokers. Although 70% of smokers say they are "interested" in quitting, only 10% to 20% plan to quit in the next month (Etter, Perneger, & Ronchi, 1997; see Table 10.2). About 45% of smokers will try to quit in a given year (Giovino et al., 1995).

In the past, 90% to 95% of smokers quit on their own. However, with the introduction of over-the-counter nicotine gum and patches, and of non-nicotine therapies, about one third of smokers now use a medication when they try to stop (Hughes, in press). In fact, most smokers use a stepwise approach to smoking cessation. They may first try to stop on their own one or more times. Then, they may use booklets or an over-the-counter (OTC) medication. Next, they may try group therapy or they may see a clinician for a prescription.

When smokers try to stop, relapse occurs quickly (Hughes et al., 1992). In those who try to quit on their own, only half succeed for 2 days and only a third last 1 week (Hughes et al., 1992). Overall, self-quitters have a success rate of 5% to 10%. Although these statistics seem discouraging, most smokers make five to seven quit attempts before they finally succeed. Thus, half of all smokers eventually quit (Giovino et al., 1995).

One implication of these statistics is that clinicians need to understand that their role is not so much helping with one quit attempt, but rather helping the smoker through several attempts before a final successful one. The other implication is that clinicians need to prompt and re-prompt smokers to make efforts to stop. Offering treatment can not only help smokers stop, but can also motivate smokers to try to stop (Shiffman et al., 1997).

TABLE 10.2. Important Statistics About Smoking Cessation

- 50% of current smokers will die from smoking if they do not quit.[a]
- Cancers of the colon, lung, stomach, and esophagus have been associated with smoking.
- Stopping smoking decreases the risk of myocardial infarction by 50% in the first year alone. Cancer risk decreases to near normal within 15 years.[a]
- Although 70% of smokers want to stop, only 35% to 45% try to quit in any given year.[b]
- Only 10% to 20% of smokers are ready to stop in the next month.[c]
- Among self-quitters, 50% remain abstinent for two days and 33% for a week.[d]
- For any given quit attempt without therapy, 5% to 10% quit for good.[d]
- Most smokers make five to seven attempts before they stop successfully; thus, 50% of smokers eventually quit smoking.[b]

[a]U.S. Department of Health and Human Services (1990).
[b]Giovino et al. (1995).
[c]Etter et al. (1997).
[d]Hughes et al. (1992).

SOME BASIC FACTS ABOUT TREATMENT

1. The efficacy of several smoking cessation therapies is well established (Table 10.3; Smoking Cessation, 1996; Hughes et al., 1996). All proven treatments appear to be equally effective: They all double the chances that a quit attempt will be successful (Table 10.4). None have significant side effects.

   Given these facts and the AHCPR guidelines, all smokers interested in quitting smoking should be encouraged to use medications. Currently, there is anecdotal experience but no proven method for matching particular treatments to particular types of smokers. In fact, early evidence suggests that allowing smokers to choose their own

TABLE 10.3. Proven Smoking Cessation Therapies

Medications	Availability
Nicotine Gum	OTC
Nicotine Patch	OTC
Nicotine Nasal Spray	Rx
Nicotine Inhaler	Rx
Bupropion	Rx
Psychosocial Therapy	
Behavior Therapy	Group or Individual

OTC = over the counter (without prescription); Rx = available by prescription only

TABLE 10.4. Typical Long-Term Quit Rates

	No Therapy	Brief Advice	Behavior Therapy
No medication or placebo	5%	10%	15%
Medication	10%	20%	30%

type of treatment produces better outcomes (American Psychiatric Association, 1998). In light of these findings, clinicians are encouraged to provide smokers with information about the proven therapies and treatment resources (Table 10.1). The American Psychiatric Association (1998), the American Lung Association (1998), and the American Cancer Society have developed consumer brochures for smokers that outline the pros and cons of the various treatments for smoking and list treatment resources.

2. With other types of drug dependencies, many experts believe psychosocial or self-help therapies are essential and that medication alone is ineffective. This is not the case, however, with nicotine dependence. For example, OTC products such as nicotine gum and patches double quit rates when used without psychosocial therapy (Hughes, 1995b; see Table 10.4). Thus, although adding psychosocial therapy certainly increases quit rates, insistence on adjunctive talk therapy as a condition for receiving prescription medication is not based on scientific evidence.

3. Although most clinicians believe that abrupt cessation is more effective than gradual nicotine reduction, empirical data to support this belief are limited (Cinciripini et al., 1995). Patients with a strong preference for gradual reduction should be allowed to use this option. They should be advised, however, not to use a nicotine replacement therapy (NRT) until they have stopped smoking completely. Switching to low tar/low nicotine cigarettes as an approach to reducing nicotine consumption does not appear to produce significant health benefit (National Cancer Institute, 1996). Finally, when dealing with smokers who are ambivalent about quitting, it is unclear that aiming for an initial goal of reducing smoking will improve health or will eventually result in smoking cessation (Hughes, 1995a).

4. Written materials, such as short motivational brochures that can be obtained from several sources (Table 10.1), should be available as handouts for patients who smoke. A list of local treatment resources is another type of handout that can be helpful.

5. Given that for most smokers, relapse occurs quickly (Hughes et al.,

1992), the first follow-up contact should be 2 to 3 days, not 1 to 2 weeks, after the quit date. This follow-up can be done via telephone or by a paraprofessional.

6. Recent evidence indicates co-morbid depression and alcohol/drug abuse are important causes for treatment failure. Cessation of smoking may, in a small minority, exacerbate these problems (Hughes, 1999). Thus, smokers with current or past histories of these problems need to be followed closely during cessation attempts.

7. Many smokers, especially women, are concerned about weight gain. Restricting food intake while trying to stop smoking worsens smoking outcomes (Perkins, 1994). Most clinicians recommend increasing physical activity or using NRT or bupropion to minimize initial postcessation weight gain (at least while therapy is used) and not attempting caloric restriction until several months after stopping smoking (Perkins, 1994).

8. The cost of medication therapy is about $3 to $4 a day, whereas fees for behavioral therapy vary from no cost to $150 or more per course of therapy. Health plans vary considerably with regard to covered services and medications.

9. Non-nicotine substances in tobacco increase the metabolism of many common drugs, such as theophylline and some antidepressants (Schein, 1995). Thus, the levels of these medications may need to be decreased with cessation. Nicotine replacement itself does not affect levels of these medications.

10. Some of the smokers requesting help from clinicians will have failed all the therapies typically used. Other smokers may have special problems, such as a sabotaging spouse or co-worker. Clinicians should identify a local psychologist, addiction counselor, other clinician, health educator, or other person with expertise in smoking cessation therapy for referral of smokers who appear to need specialized help (Table 10.1).

11. Clinicians can learn more about smoking cessation therapies from a variety of sources, such as short articles (Hughes et al., 1999) and books (Hughes, 1996). In addition, they can attend annual educational meetings held by the American Society of Addiction Medicine and the Society for Research on Nicotine and Tobacco (Table 10.1).

WHAT'S NEW ABOUT OLD TREATMENTS?

Between 1995 and 1996, nicotine gum and two of the four currently approved nicotine patches became available without prescription. Several studies conducted in OTC settings confirmed that the use of gum or patch doubled cessation rates with no evidence of significant adverse events (Hughes et al., 1999).

The availability of nicotine gum and transdermal patches without prescription has produced the largest increase in smoking cessation since the 1964 Surgeon General's report on smoking (Hughes, in press).

Clinicians often recommend or are asked about OTC treatments and this is clearly true for nicotine patches and gum. Since these products were originally marketed, much information has continued to accrue, further enhancing and documenting the efficacy and safety of such therapies. For example, there are no longer any true contraindications to the use of these products in smokers. Almost all researchers agree that nicotine is not a carcinogen (Benowitz, 1998), and there is growing consensus that nicotine derived from medications does not promote cardiovascular disease (Benowitz & Gourlay, 1997). Finally, in addition to the fact that gum and patch formulations are associated with a slower onset and much lower nicotine levels than are cigarettes, they do not produce carbon monoxide and carcinogens (Hughes, 1996). Consistent with these findings, the safety and abuse liability records of nicotine gum and patches have been excellent (Murray et al., 1996).

The OTC labeling on nicotine gum and patches instructs smokers to see their clinicians before using the products if they have heart disease, ulcers, or uncontrolled hypertension. This recommendation is made because clinicians may wish to monitor these patients' progress more closely when such individuals stop smoking.

Labeling also directs smokers who are pregnant or breastfeeding to see their healthcare providers before using nicotine gum or patch. How much of the harm associated with smoking during pregnancy is due to nicotine, carbon monoxide, or other substances is unclear (Hughes, 1993). Clearly, the fetus is exposed to much less nicotine with gum or patches than with smoking. Most reviews recommend that nicotine gum or a patch be considered for smoking cessation in those pregnant smokers who want to quit but have failed nonnicotine therapies (Hughes, 1993).

The OTC labels recommend not using nicotine gum or patches along with other nicotine products. However, three studies have found that the combined use of a nicotine patch plus 2 mg nicotine gum ad lib (usually four to eight pieces/day used during craving episodes) increases quit rates by 6% to 7% over either product alone with no increase in side effects (Hughes, 1999). Thus, many smoking cessation specialists recommend that patients use a patch plus gum ad lib for "high craving situations."

Another labeled warning that has recently been shown not to be a concern is about smoking while using the patch. An initial small case series suggested that smoking while wearing a patch could cause myocardial infarctions. Several well-controlled studies in patients with active heart disease have shown, however, that this is not true (Benowitz, 1998). In fact, a recent study tested smokers wearing a triple-dose nicotine patch (63 mg/day) while smoking 15 cigarettes/day and found no evidence of cardiovascular problems (Zevin, Jacobs, & Benowitz, 1998).

PRESCRIPTION NICOTINE REPLACEMENT

Nicotine Nasal Spray

The nicotine nasal spray was designed to rapidly administer higher levels of replacement nicotine. Although it does deliver larger doses more rapidly than nicotine gum and patches, the delivery rate and magnitude are still much lower than those of cigarettes (Schneider et al., 1996). And while the nasal spray also doubles quit rates (Hughes, 1999), whether it is superior to gum or patches is unknown.

The spray causes nasal and throat irritation, rhinitis, sneezing, coughing, and lacrimation in the large majority of smokers during the first week of use, although tolerance occurs rapidly. Early concerns about the dependence liability of the spray have not been borne out (Hughes, 1999). Although unconfirmed by trials, nasal spray might be best for smokers who appear to need large doses of nicotine.

Nicotine Inhaler

The nicotine inhaler is a plastic rod containing a plug impregnated with nicotine. It is designed to combine pharmacological and behavioral substitution strategies. When warm air passes over the plug, nicotine vapor is produced. Although described as an inhaler, in actuality, nicotine from the device is absorbed buccally, rather than in the lungs (Bergstrom et al., 1995). The pharmacokinetics and blood levels of nicotine that result from the "inhaler" are similar, therefore, to those seen with nicotine gum.

This device appears to be helpful for those who desire a behavioral substitute for cigarettes. However, the efficacy of the inhaler is not due solely to behavioral replacement, as active-ingredient inhalers double quit rates compared with placebo inhalers (Hughes, 1999). Side effects from the inhaler include mild mouth and throat irritation and coughing. Dependence on the device has not been a significant problem (Hughes, 1999). The nicotine inhaler loses some bioavailability at temperatures below 10° C.

NON-NICOTINE MEDICATIONS

Many smokers prefer a non-nicotine medication, and many have failed in previous efforts to quit using NRT.

Bupropion

This medication is an atypical antidepressant that doubles quit rates (Hughes, 1999). It is prescribed as 300 mg/day of the slow-release preparation, beginning 1 week prior to the quit date (Hurt et al., 1997). Importantly, bupropion does not appear to work via its antidepressant effects; that is, it is effective in those with no current or past depressive symptoms (Goldstein, 1998).

The most common side effects of bupropion are dry mouth and insomnia (Goldstein, 1998). Seizure risk appears to be minimal with use of the slow-release preparation, doses less than or equal to 300 mg/day, and with appropriate screening for a history of seizures, anorexia, heavy alcohol use, or head trauma (Goldstein, 1998). There are no adequate and well-controlled studies in pregnant women. One study found that combining bupropion and a nicotine patch increased short-term quit rates somewhat over bupropion used alone (Goldstein, 1998). Recent trials have suggested that some other antidepressants (e.g., nortriptyline) might be helpful (Hall et al., 1998; Prochazka et al., 1998), whereas others (e.g., fluoxetine) do not appear to be beneficial.

Clonidine

Clonidine is an alpha-2 antagonist that has also been shown to double quit rates (Gourlay & Benowitz, 1995). However, the evidence of its efficacy is less robust and it appears to have more side effects (postural hypotension, drowsiness, etc.) than other medications (Gourlay & Benowitz, 1995). Clonidine is usually used only as a second-line medication.

PSYCHOSOCIAL THERAPIES

Behavioral therapy is the only proven psychosocial treatment for smoking cessation (Hughes et al., 1996; Smoking Cessation, 1996), doubling quit rates (Smoking Cessation, 1996). Usually administered in a group setting so that smokers also receive social support, it can also be conducted on an individual basis. The major disadvantage of behavior therapy has not been its efficacy but rather its limited availability and acceptability. For example, although several organizations offer behavior therapy (Table 10.1), in most communities, groups are run only 2 or 3 times a year. Thus, if a smoker is ready to stop and wants to try group therapy, he or she often has to wait months for a group to become available. In the meantime, the motivation to stop smoking may diminish. Individual therapy is also often unavailable or, if it is available, is costly due to lack of insurance coverage.

On the other hand, all of the medications discussed here have telephone-based behavior therapy programs that are offered free to interested smokers. At least one study suggests that, although the amount of interpersonal contact in these programs is limited, they still increase quit rates by tailoring therapy to the smoker's specific problems (Shiffman et al., 2001).

Written materials are often used with both medication and behavioral therapies. Although they do not appear effective when used on their own, they are thought to improve outcomes of other therapies (Curry, 1993).

SUMMARY

Many clinicians still approach smoking interventions as unpleasant interactions involving cajoling, berating, or pleading with patients. With the advent of several proven effective therapies, smoking interventions should instead be viewed as potentially positive interactions in which the clinician can offer support and concrete help to smokers. If even a few patients can be convinced and helped to quit, the practitioner will have made a major contribution to his or her patients' overall health and longevity.

REFERENCES

American Lung Association. (1998). *Quit smoking action plan.* New York: Author.

American Psychiatric Association. (1998). *Treatment works: When you choose to stop smoking.* Washington DC: Author.

Benowitz, N. L., & Gourlay, S. G. (1997). Cardiovascular toxicity of nicotine: Implications for nicotine replacement therapy. *Journal of the American College of Cardiology, 29,* 1422–1431.

Benowitz, N. L. (1998). *Nicotine safety and toxicity.* New York: Oxford University Press.

Bergstrom, M., Nordberg, A., Lunell, E., et al. (1995). Regional deposition of inhaled 11C-nicotine vapor in the human airway as visualized by positron emission tomography. *Clinical Pharmacology and Therapeutics, 57,* 309–317.

Cinciripini, P. M., Lapitsky, L., Seay, S., et al. (1995). The effects of smoking schedules on cessation outcome: Can we improve on common methods of gradual and abrupt nicotine withdrawal? *Journal of Consulting and Clinical Psychology, 63,* 388–399.

Cromwell, J., Bartosch, W. J., Fiore, M. C., et al. (1997). Cost-effectiveness of the clinical practice recommendations in the AHCPR Guideline for Smoking Cessation. *Journal of the American Medical Association, 278,* 1759–1766.

Curry, S. J. (1993). Self-help interventions for smoking cessation. *Journal of Consulting and Clinical Psychology, 61,* 790–803.

Etter, J. F., Perneger, T. V., & Ronchi, A. (1997). Distributions of smokers by stage: International comparison and association with smoking prevalence. *Preventive Medicine, 26,* 580–585.

Fagerstrom, K.-O., Tejding, R., Ake, W., et al. (1997). Aiding reduction of smoking with nicotine replacement medications: Hope for the recalcitrant smoker? *Tobacco Control, 6,* 311–316.

Giovino, G. A., Henningfield, J. E., Tomar, S. L., et al. (1995). Epidemiology of tobacco use and dependence. *Epidemiologic Reviews, 17,* 48–65.

Glynn, T. J., & Manley, M. W. (1989). *How to help your patients stop smoking.* Washington, DC: U.S. Government Printing Office.

Goldstein, M. G. (1998). Bupropion sustained release and smoking cessation. *Journal of Clinical Psychiatrry, 59* (suppl. 4), 66–72.

Gourlay, S. G., & Benowitz, N. L. (1995). Is clonidine an effective smoking cessation therapy? *Drugs, 50,* 197–207.

Hall, S. M., Reus, V. I., Munoz, R. F., et al. (1998). Nortriptyline and cognitive-behavioral therapy in the treatment of cigarette smoking. *Archives of General Psychiatry, 55,* 683–690.

Hughes, J. R. (1993). Risk/benefit of nicotine replacement in smoking cessation. *Drug Safety, 8,* 49–56.

Hughes, J. R. (1995a). Applying harm reduction to smoking. *Tobacco Control, 4,* S33–S38.

Hughes, J, R. (1995b). Combining behavioral therapy and pharmacotherapy for smoking cessation: An update. In L. S. Onken, J. D. Blaine, & J. J. Boren (Eds.), *Integrating behavior therapies with medication in the treatment of drug dependence* (pp. 92–109). NIDA Research Monograph 150. Washington, DC: U.S. Government Printing Office.

Hughes, J. R. (1996). Pharmacotherapy of nicotine dependence. In C. R. Schuster & M. J. Kuhar (Eds.), *Pharmacological aspects of drug dependence: Toward an integrative neurobehavioral approach, handbook of experimental pharmacology series* (pp. 599–626). New York: Springer-Verlag.

Hughes, J. R. (1999). Comorbidity and smoking. *Nicotine and Tobacco Research, 1,* S149–S152.

Hughes, J. R. (in press). Impact of medications on smoking cessation. In D. Burns (Ed.), *Population impact of smoking cessation interventions.* NCI Monograph.

Hughes, J. R., Fiester, S., Goldstein, M. G., et al. (1996). American Psychiatric Association practice guideline for the treatment of patients with nicotine dependence. *American Journal of Psychiatrry, 153,* S1–31.

Hughes, J. R., Goldstein, M. G., Hurt, R. D., et al. (1999). Recent advances in pharmacotherapy of smoking. *Journal of the American Medical Association, 281,* 72–76.

Hughes, J. R., Gulliver, S. B., Fenwick, J. W., et al. (1992). Smoking cessation among self-quitters. *Health Psychology, 11,* 331–334.

Hurt, R. D., Sachs, D., Glover, E. D., et al. (1997). A comparison of sustained-release bupropion and placebo for smoking cessation. *New England Journal of Medicine, 337,* 1195–1202.

Murray, R. P., Bailey, W. C., Daniels, K., et al. (1996). Safety of nicotine polacrilex gum used by 3,094 participants in the Lung Health Study. *Chest, 109,* 438–445.

National Cancer Institute Expert Committee: (1996). *The FTC cigarette test method for determining tar, nicotine and carbon monoxide yields of U.S. cigarettes.* Smoking and Tobacco Control Monograph #7, Bethesda, MD: National Cancer Institute.

Perkins, K. A. (1994). Issues in the prevention of weight gain after smoking cessation. *Annals of Behavioral Medicine, 16,* 46–52.

Prochazka, A. V., Weaver, M. J., Keller, R. T., et al. (1998). A randomized trial of nortriptyline for smoking cessation. *Archives of Internal Medicine, 58,* 2035–2039.

Schein, J. R. (1995). Cigarette smoking and clinically significant drug interactions. *Annals of Pharmacotherapy, 29,* 1139–1148.

Schneider, N. G., Lunell, E., Olmstead, R. E., et al. (1996). Clinical pharmacokinetics of nasal nicotine delivery: A review and comparison to other nicotine systems. *Clinical Pharmacokinetics, 31,* 65–80.

Shiffman, S., Paty, J. A., Rohay, J., et al. (2001). The efficacy of computer-tailored smoking cessation material as a supplement to nicotine patch therapy. *Drug and Alcohol Dependency, 64*(1), 35–46.

Shiffman, S., Pinney, J. M., Gitchell, J., et al. (1997). Public health benefit of over-the-counter nicotine medications. *Tobacco Control,* 306–310.

Smoking Cessation Clinical Practice Guideline Panel and Staff. (1996). The Agency for Health Care Policy and Research Smoking Cessation Clinical Practice Guideline 18. *Journal of the American Medical Association, 275,* 1270–1280.

U.S. Department of Health and Human Services. (1990). *Health benefits of smoking cessation. A report of the U.S. Surgeon General.* Rockville, MD: Author.

Zevin, S., Jacob, III P., & Benowitz, N. (1998). Dose-related cardiovascular and endocrine effects of transdermal nicotine. *Clinical Pharmacology and Therapeutics, 64,* 87–95.

Permission Acknowledgments

The following articles were previously published. Permission to reprint is gratefully acknowledged here.

Carroll, Kathleen M. (1999). Old psychotherapies for cocaine dependence revisited. *Archives of General Psychiatry, 56*(6), 505–506. Copyright © 1999 American Medical Association.

Glanz, Morton, Klawansky, Sidney, McAuliffe, William, & Chalmers, Thomas. (1997) Methadone vs. L-alpha-acetylmethadol (LAAM) in the treatment of opiate addiction: A meta-analysis of the randomized, controlled trials. *The American Journal on Addictions, 6*(4), 339–349. Copyright © 1997 American Academy of Addiction Psychiatry. Reprinted by permission of Brunner-Routledge and Taylor and Francis.

Holder, Harold D., Cisler, Ron A., Longabaugh, Richard, Stout, Robert L., Treno, Andrew J., & Zweben, Allen. (2000). Alcoholism treatment and medical care costs from Project MATCH. *Addiction, 95*(7), 999–1013. Copyright © Society for the Study of Addiction to Alcohol and Other Drugs. Reprinted by permission of Carfax Publishing and Taylor and Francis.

Hughes, John R. (2000). New treatments for smoking cessation. *CA—Cancer Journal for Clinicians, 50*(3), 143–151; quiz, 152–155. Reprinted by permission of the publisher.

Kosten, Thomas R. (1998). The pharmacotherapy of relapse prevention using anticonvulsants. *The American Journal on Addictions, 7*(3), 205–209. Copyright © 1998 American Academy of Addiction Psychiatry. Reprinted by permission of Brunner-Routledge and Taylor and Francis.

Litten, Raye Z., & Allen, John P. (1999). Medications for alcohol, illicit drug, and tobacco dependence: An update of research finding*s. Journal of Substance Abuse Treatment, 16*(2), 105–112. Copyright © 1999 Elsevier Science Inc. Reprinted by permission.

O'Connor, Patrick G., & Fiellin, David A. (2000). Pharmacologic treatment of heroin-dependent patients. *Annals of Internal Medicine, 133*(1), 40–54. Copyright © American College of Physicians—American Society of Internal Medicine. Reprinted by permission of the American College of Physicians—American Society of Internal Medicine.

Pages, Kenneth P., & Ries, Richard K. (1998). Use of anticonvulsants in benzodiazepine withdrawal. *The American Journal on Addictions, 7,* 198–204. Copyright © 1998 The American Academy of Addiction Psychiatry. Reprinted by permission of Brunner-Routledge and Taylor and Francis.

Siqueland, Lynne, & Crits-Christoph, Paul. (1999). Current developments in psychosocial treatments of alcohol and substance sbuse. *Current Psychiatry Reports, 1*(2), 179–184. Copyright © 1999 Current Science Inc. Reprinted by permission conveyed through the Copyright Clearance Center, Inc.

Swift, Robert M. (1999). Drug therapy for alcohol dependence. *New England Journal of Medicine, 340,* 1482–1490. Copyright © 1999 Massachusetts Medical Society. All rights reserved. Reprinted by permission of the Massachusetts Medical Society.

Index

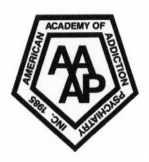

About the American Academy of Addiction Psychiatry

The American Academy of Addiction Psychiatry (AAAP) is a professional membership organization with approximately 1,000 members in the United States and around the world. The membership consists of health professionals who work with addiction in their practices, faculty at various academic institutions, residents, and medical students.

The AAAP was founded in 1985:

- to promote accessibility to highest quality treatment for all who need it,
- to promote excellence in clinical practice in addiction psychiatry,
- to educate the public and influence public policy regarding addictive illness,
- to provide continuing education for addiction professionals,
- to disseminate new information in the field of addiction psychiatry,
- to encourage research on the etiology, prevention, identification, and treatment of the addictions.

AAAP sponsors various scientific meetings, including an Annual Scientific Meeting and Symposium, a Review Course on Addiction Psychiatry, and symposia and workshops on timely clinical, educational, and research topics in the addiction field.

The American Journal on Addictions, a leading clinical journal listed in *Index Medicus* and many other databases, is the official journal of AAAP. The journal serves as a forum from which today's leading clinicians gain rapid access to advances in current treatment methods, original peer-reviewed research, and improved clinical outcome.

For more information about AAAP activities or to request a membership packet, call 913-262-6161, e-mail info@aaap.org, or visit the AAAP Web site, www.aaap.org.